医学英语学术交流教程

Medical English
for Academic Communication

主　编　丁春生　王栩彬

副主编　王　然　李　平

编　委（以姓氏拼音排序）

程　炯　丁春生　计红丽

李　平　李雪梅　刘　军

刘维静　王　然　王栩彬

王燕茹　徐　燕　张禄静

朱蕾蔓

 南京大学出版社

图书在版编目(CIP)数据

医学英语学术交流教程 / 丁春生,王栩彬主编. —
南京:南京大学出版社,2019.9
ISBN 978 - 7 - 305 - 22477 - 5

Ⅰ. ①医… Ⅱ. ①丁… ②王… Ⅲ. ①医学—英语—
医学院校—教材 Ⅳ. ①R

中国版本图书馆 CIP 数据核字(2019)第 149616 号

出版发行　南京大学出版社
社　　址　南京市汉口路 22 号　　　　邮　编　210093
出 版 人　金鑫荣
书　　名　医学英语学术交流教程
主　　编　丁春生　王栩彬
责任编辑　裴维维　　　　　　　　　编辑热线　025 - 83592123
照　　排　南京南琳图文制作有限公司
印　　刷　丹阳兴华印务有限公司
开　　本　787×1092　1/16　印张 13.25　字数 390 千
版　　次　2019 年 9 月第 1 版　2019 年 9 月第 1 次印刷
ISBN 978 - 7 - 305 - 22477 - 5
定　　价　47.00 元

网址:http://www.njupco.com
官方微博:http://weibo.com/njupco
南大悦学:njuyuexue
销售咨询热线:(025) 83594756

前　言

经历了多年的学习和淬炼,高年级医学本科同学及硕、博士们都具备了很强的英语文献阅读能力和英语论文写作能力,所欠缺的外语能力主要体现在学术口语交际以及西方文化认知等方面。随着其学术研究的深入,以及国际化和全球化进程的加快,他们会越来越多地参与国际学术交流,这使得上述外语能力缺陷的表现越发明显,相关需求日益突出。

针对相关同学对外语学习的上述需求,我们根据本校高年级英语教学实践,编写了《医学英语学术交流教程》。本书共 8 个单元。每个单元均包含视听说、阅读和口语三部分。

视听说选取各种国际会议和学术交流的音视频资料,帮助学生提升听力水平;设计相关问题,提供学生进行口语表达的机会。

阅读文章 2 篇:Text A 为精读材料,Text B 为泛读材料。材料均选自国际医学学术期刊、书籍或权威医学网站上的英文文章,强化学生的文献阅读能力、提升词汇学习效率的同时,通过课后练习,引入 group discussion 和 oral presentation,让学生能就问题展开讨论并独立表达观点。

口语分为:1. 临床问诊英语口语,以诊室语境为背景,提高学生英语问诊能力;2. 国际会议英语口语,以国际学术会议为纲,涉及会议整个流程中需要的英语内容;3. 向西方介绍中国,从跨文化交际的角度出发,在国际会议和交流中向西方人介绍中国人的思想和文化特点,让世界更了解中国。

在体例、内容和编排上,我们淡化了低年级本科生医学英语里重视的语法、句法、医学词汇构词法以及医学文献阅读等方面内容,也弱化了文献阅读以及论文写作等方面能力的内容,而是着重强调学术口语交际能力和跨文化交际能力的培养,以及文化认知、文化对比等方面的知识的储备和意识的树立。

以诱导讨论式教学法和 TBL(Team-Based Learning)教学模式为基调,在本书的编写过程中,我们处处重视对学术口语及跨文化交际能力的培养。Oral presentation 和 group discussion 练习的设计,使得学生们在课堂上就能获得大量的机会来亲身感受国际学术活动的氛围,锻炼自己的口语表达能力,提升跨文化交际水平。口语部分中,临床问诊英语口语的设计,意在锻炼学生英语问诊能力;国际会议口语部分,从报名参会到会议流程设计,从会议接待到主持发言,从会议报告到宴会祝酒,意在提升学生在参加和主办国际学术会议时,以更流畅的交流,取得更大的收获。

古来大医皆大儒。只顾着提高医疗技术,忽视了文化修养的提升,无法成为真正伟大的医生。作为一门艺术,任何医学和产生该门医学的文化都密不可分。很难想象一位对阴阳五行学说没有深入研究的人能成为名符其实的中医,同样,将产生于西方的现代医学与其文化土壤割裂开来,医学将彻底沦为机械操作,医生也因失去精神支撑和文化滋润,终难成就大医。为此,本书专门设置了文化部分,在口语交际中提升学生们对文化的深层认知。添上这个环节,补齐文化短板,使得他们能够用技术与文化两条腿走路,均衡发展,两翼齐飞。另外,本书还通过对艺术、宗教、生活方式和山川地貌等各方面进行介绍和对比,旨在培养学生的国际视野和文化意识。用西方人的思想和理念去理解西方先进科技的发展;用东方人的哲学和方式去"师夷长技"并因地制宜地将其应用和发展,提高我们的技术水平;用跨文化的意识去进行交流,去学习他们的成果,去推广我们的文化。

付印之前,本书已在安徽医科大学进行课堂教学实践,取得了良好的教学互动和教学效果,并对反映出来的相关不足之处进行了修改。

本书的策划和编写由安徽医科大学人文医学学院和外语系直接领导,过程中得到了省内多家著名医院以及高校外语学院(系)专家和领导们的关心、指导和帮助,在此致以衷心感谢。

虽然编者努力想给大家奉献一本好书,但囿于学识浅薄,疏漏之处在所难免。我们殷切希望广大师生在使用过程中提出宝贵意见,以便我们不断修订和改进,使之更臻完善。

编　者
2019 年 9 月

Contents

Unit 8

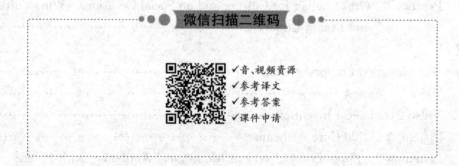

Unit 1

Key Points

Learning Targets
- To master the listening skill of *Prediction*
- To improve the reading skill of *Skimming*
- To learn about the academic terms of cardiology in clinical diagnostic conversation

Learning Focus
- How to declare the beginning and ending of an international academic conference
- How to register for an international conference

Cultural Points
- Chinese dining culture

✓音、视频资源
✓参考译文
✓参考答案
✓学术探讨

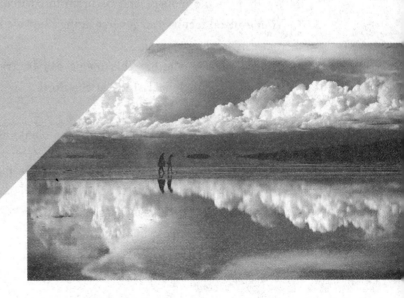

Part Ⅰ Listening Comprehension

Video 1

How Young Blood Might Help Reverse Aging

Exercise Ⅰ Watch the video and decide whether the following statements are true (T) or false (F).

1. The speaker is going to show some factors that can modulate the age of a tissue.
2. Parabiosis is done in mice by surgically connecting the two mice together, which then leads to a shared neural system.
3. We've reasoned that it must be the soluble factor—plasma in blood could reproduce these rejuvenating effects.
4. In the memory test, the old mouse with memory problems just looks into every hole, but it doesn't form the spacial map to support its escape.
5. In the memory test, another young mouse looks around and then walks straight to that hole and escapes.
6. We find the old mouse, and its brain in particular, can be changed and reshaped.
7. Young blood factors can reverse aging, but we haven't found any old blood factors that can accelerate aging.
8. In order to see whether this magic can be transferable to other animals, we're running a small clinical study at Stanford.

Exercise Ⅱ Watch the video and fill in the blanks in the note.

Findings through Parabiosis
A. More 9. _____
B. 10. _____ of the synapses, 11. _____
C. More genes involved in 12. _____
D. Less of 13. _____

Video 2 ▌▌▌▌▌

Cancer Genomics and Precision Medicine in the 21st Century

Exercise Ⅰ   Take notes while watching the video and fill in the blanks in the table.

Changes in View of Lung Cancer	
Traditional view	1.
In 1987	2.
In 2004	3.
In 2009	HER 2 over expressions, BRAF mutations, metal alterations, some AKT, some PIC3CA, or PI3 kinase mutations.

Exercise Ⅱ   Take notes while watching the video and fill in the blanks in the table.

The Shifting Paradigm in Medicine	
Previous approaches	New practices
Descriptive medicine	4.
Empiric diagnosis	5.
Grouped by organ site	6.
7.	Individualized treatment
Retrospectively diagnosea disease	Prospectively intervene
Acute care	8.

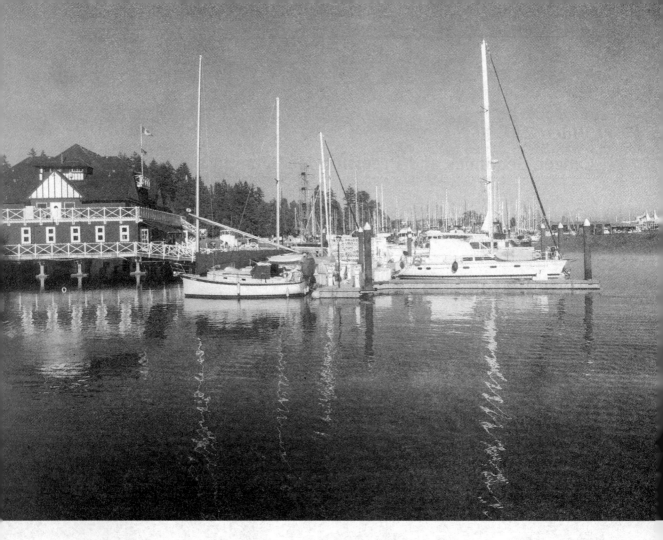

Exercise Ⅲ Watch the video and answer the following questions.

9. What is the speaker's field of research?
10. What does the speaker mean by descriptive medicine?
11. What does the speaker prefer to call individualized therapy?
12. How can we select drugs according to the speaker?
13. What have we thought of cancer for many years?

Exercise Ⅳ Take notes and fill in the blanks.

a. Founder mutation usually refers to 14. _____. You will see that in all tumors that are biopsied. And then there are often lesions that lead to 15. _____, like P53, which is called 16. _____. So one of the problems is many of these founder mutations 17. _____. And they are often not 18. _____.

b. What we mean by driver mutations is that those are required for the expression of 19. _____. And the driver mutations are those that we think we should be able to 20. _____ and then successfully 21. _____.

Listening 1 ||||

The Prevention of Cancer

Exercise I   Listen to the speech and decide whether the following statements are true (T) or false (F).

1. The speaker mainly talks about infectious causes of cancer in this part of the speech.
2. Occupational cancers vary over history depending on contemporary industries.
3. One of the earliest recognized occupational cancers was scrotal cancer.
4. Around 4 percent of the UK cancers are due to occupation and are relatively straight-forwardly preventable in an economically viable way.
5. The major occupational cancers tend to be skin cancer, sinonasal cancer and larynx one.
6. Cancers are completely preventable, especially those from infectious reasons.

Exercise II   Please arrange the following risk factors of cancer in the right order according to the list mentioned in the speech.

| A. diesel exhaust | B. radon | C. silica dust |
| D. mineral oils | E. asbestos | F. paint |

7. No. 1 _____
8. No. 2 _____
9. No. 3 _____
10. No. 4 _____
11. No. 5 _____
12. No. 6 _____

Exercise III   Listen to the speech and fill in the blanks.

a. The speaker chose mesothelioma as an example. It is an extremely unpleasant 13. _____, which is very difficult to treat, also 14. _____. About 95% of the risk is related to 15. _____, and almost all of that is 16. _____.

b. The cancer rates have been 17. _____ and only peaked in the last few years, although we've stopped now using asbestos and it's much more heavily regulated. They will now steadily decline because 18. _____ and sadly because many people who are exposed are dying of mesothelioma.

Listening 2
Using Risk Models for Breast Cancer Prevention

Exercise Ⅰ Classify the following risk factors into different groups.

A. strong risk factor   B. moderately strong risk factor   C. weak risk factor

1. Age
2. Age at first birth
3. Age at menarche
4. Age at menopause
5. Adverse SNP in FGFR2
6. BRCA 1 or BRCA 2
7. BMI
8. Contralateral breast cancer
9. Drinking ethanol
10. Family history
11. Having biopsies
12. Hormone replacement therapy
13. Mammographic density
14. Radiation
15. Western country

Exercise Ⅱ Listen to the speech and fill in the blanks in the note.

Some Choices in Risk Modeling

A. Based on 16. _____ or empirical approach
B. Choice of risk factors
  a. Detailed or only some 17. _____
  b. Reproductive history
  c. Medical history factors (e. g. biopsies, 18. _____)
C. 19. _____ in the models and how to piece together
D. 20. _____ : e. g. general population in the UK or the US; or 21. _____

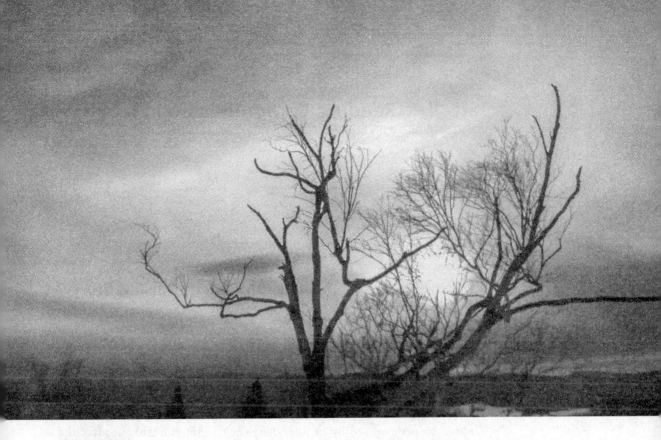

Exercise Ⅲ Listen to the speech and decide whether the following statements are true (T) or false (F).

22. The speaker gives some examples of models based on empirical approach.
23. Some of the models were based on the assumption that breast cancer is an autosomal dominant disease.
24. BRCAPRO, a widely used model, allows us to use extensive family history without any mutation data.
25. Elizabeth did a study herself which showed that really familial aggregation patterns of breast cancer can be explained entirely by autosomal dominance.
26. BRCA genes only account for 20 percent of the familial aggregation.
27. Others have tried to expand on the autosomal dominant model by considering residual familial correlations beyond those ascribed to the dominant mutations.

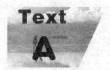

Nutrition in Public Health: An Unfinished Story

José Maria Bengoa

I often recall past times. Almost 60 years ago, in 1948, 60 professionals with a commitment to launch the fight against malnutrition in Latin America met in Montevideo. From the fifties to the seventies, the central theme of international meetings was kwashiorkor caused by protein deficiency. This came about after the seminal publication by Cicely Williams of an article with the strange name of "kwashiorkor". Only a few years later it was revealed that in a local language in Ghana it meant "the disease of the first son when the second is born". It was Cicely Williams' suggestion that the treatment was protein-rich skim milk. It was believed that the fundamental cause of kwashiorkor was protein deficiency, which is why many meetings focused on the issue of the "protein gap".

When FAO and WHO were created, one of the first objectives to which considerable resources were allocated was to look for new nonconventional sources of protein, in cooperation with UNICEF. The best centers related to nutritional investigation started to develop new protein-rich formulas with the objective of providing much-needed relief to developing countries.

Today the issue appears somewhat different, and what is outstanding is chronic protein-energy malnutrition, with its major consequence of small size.

Changes in lifestyles

One could argue that in the future there will be substantial changes in lifestyle, changes that are already visible and are modeling the alimentary traditions. We are advancing toward a uniform way of eating worldwide, such that traditional foods and dishes of many populations will probably be maintained only in rural areas. Some of the most valuable signs of identity will thus be lost. Only 10 or 12 foodstuffs will dominate international commerce. Time dedicated to meal preparation at home will shrink, and industry will take the place formerly held by the housewife.

Fast food will dominate in the cosmopolitan urban world, and it will be no different in Mexico or in Geneva. From that standpoint, one could question whether nutrition science will become easier, more homogeneous, and consequently more boring. Will we not lose the charm of those anthropological discussions about the cultural differences in nutritional traditions that have delighted us in the past? The family meal is unfortunately coming to an end, and soon enough we will pray a requiem in memoriam.

Recent studies have demonstrated the links between infant malnutrition and the rise in obesity and other chronic diseases. This thesis is based on strong scientific evidence that requires a global focus on the alimentary problems of populations. This is another great challenge for new generations.

However, these initiatives should not fall into the trap of unnecessary excesses. One such extreme case, unacceptable to any ethically conscious nutritionist, can be found in a report by a WHO Expert Committee, "Prevention and fight against cardiovascular diseases in the community." It reads, "Presently there are techniques that can remove fat from milk therefore new applications must be found for these fatty compounds so eliminated. Among these applications may be considered their use in animal foods or in the soap industry."

In a hungry world with obvious caloric deficiencies and where thousands of children become blind because of vitamin A deficiency, it appears outrageous to use butter to make soap!

All the changes, spontaneous or induced, will impact the nutritional status of populations, and although in certain cases there may be some worsening, they may also bring about more social uniformity.

Nevin Scrimshaw points out that in the 20th century good results were obtained in the following areas:
» Controlling vitamin and iodine deficiencies;
» Promoting maternal breastfeeding;

» Incorporation of folic acid and iron into supplementation programs;

» Improvement of food programs for refugees;

» Promotion of nutrition as a human right.

Nonetheless, he also stresses that some programs have been failures, including:

» Complementary nutrition—the so-called magic bullet programs to control iron deficiency.

I would like to mention as well that the 20th century has seen:

» The eradication of most vitamin deficiency diseases, with the significant exception of vitamin A deficiency;

» A remarkable increase in professionals and nongovernmental organizations (NGOs) dedicated to nutrition;

» A marked decrease in endemic goiter and cretinism;

» A careful progression in food-enrichment programs;

» Obvious progress in enteral and parenteral nutrition;

» A growing importance of community nutrition programs.

One could also add a number of other achievements in areas of health, education, and agriculture that have contributed to the improvement of the nutritional condition of populations.

Trends in nutritional indicators

Vital indicators have clearly improved over the past decades. Life expectancy has increased worldwide, reaching 66 years. Let us remember that in 1981 a goal of 60 years was established, which has now been surpassed by 6 years. Nowadays women live 6 years longer than men in developed countries and 3 years longer in developing countries. Although life expectancy at birth in developed countries is 77 years, it is still 51 years in developing countries.

A goal was established of 50 per thousand for infant mortality. Today the average value is 64 per thousand, with a range from 120 per thousand in the least developed countries to 5 per thousand in most advanced nations.

The greatest difference between developing and developed countries is seen in maternal mortality. Whereas the latter boast a rate of 10 for 100,000 live births, the former have rates of up to 100 per 100,000 live births. This index cries out the inequities in development between rich and poor countries.

Infectious diseases for which there are preventive vaccines have been considerably reduced all over the world. Despite this success, there still are more than 3 million deaths due to diseases preventable by immunization, particularly measles, which claims more than 1 million lives every year. Tuberculosis is again emerging as a major health issue, with more than 8 million new cases, 95% of them in developing countries.

As we move on from the synergy between malnutrition and infectious diseases, a favorite topic of Nevin Scrimshaw, to the new paradox of poor nutrition and obesity, new challenges for the nutrition community arise that will require further scrutiny. The history of nutrition in public health is thus an unfinished story.

(1038 words)

※ The text is extracted from the keynote address from the First World Congress on Public Health Nutrition. The author was Head of Nutrition of the World Health Organization from 1955 through 1975.

 Vocabulary

malnutrition	[ˌmælnjʊˈtrɪʃ(ə)n]	n.	营养失调,营养不良
kwashiorkor	[ˌkwɒʃɪˈɔːkɔː]	n.	夸希奥科病;恶性营养不良病
seminal	[ˈsemɪn(ə)l]	adj.	精液的;开创性的
skim milk		n.	脱脂牛奶
alimentary	[ˌælɪˈment(ə)rɪ]	adj.	饮食的;营养的
homogeneous	[ˌhɒmə(ʊ)ˈdʒiːnɪəs]	adj.	同种的;同质的
requiem	[ˈrekwɪəm]	n.	安魂曲;追思弥撒
cardiovascular	[ˌkɑːdɪəʊˈvæskjʊlə]	adj.	心血管的
spontaneous	[spɒnˈteɪnɪəs]	adj.	自发的;自然的
iodine	[ˈaɪədiːn]	n.	碘;碘酒
maternal	[məˈtɜːn(ə)l]	adj.	母亲的;母性的;母系的
folic acid	[ˈfəʊlɪk] [ˈæsɪd]	n.	叶酸,维生素B
endemic	[enˈdemɪk]	adj.	地方性的;风土的
goiter	[ˈɡɒɪtə]	n.	甲状腺肿
cretinism	[ˈkriːtɪˌnɪzəm]	n.	白痴病;呆小症
enteral	[ˈentər(ə)l]	adj.	肠的;肠内的
parenteral	[pəˈrent(ə)r(ə)l]	adj.	肠胃外的;不经肠道的
mortality	[mɔːˈtælɪtɪ]	n.	死亡数,死亡率
measles	[ˈmiːz(ə)lz]	n.	麻疹;风疹
tuberculosis	[tjʊˌbɜːkjʊˈləʊsɪs]	n.	肺结核;结核病
synergy	[ˈsɪnədʒɪ]	n.	协同作用;增效

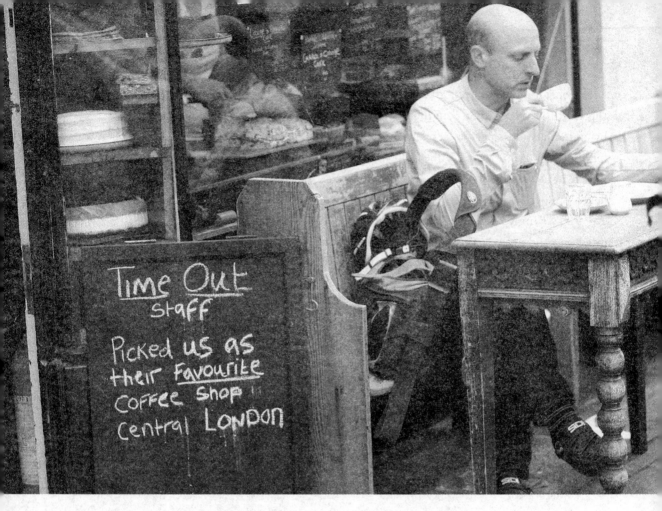

| scrutiny | [ˈskruːtɪnɪ] | n. 详细审查；监视；细看 |

◆ Questions

1. Why did many meetings focus on "protein gap" from the 1950s to the 1970s?
2. What is the outstanding issue for nutrition in public health nowadays?
3. What are the main changes modeling the alimentary traditions?
4. What are the good results obtained in public health nutrition in the 20th century?
5. What are the vital nutrition indicators mentioned in the text? And what does the difference in these indicators between developed and developing countries reflect?
6. What is the new challenge for the nutrition community?
7. Some nutritionists point out that "Obesity is also a form of malnutrition." What do you think of the paradox of malnutrition and obesity in the contemporary world? How can we prevent obesity from the perspective of nutrition?

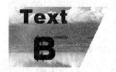

Lessons Learned in Controlling the
Burden of Malnutrition

Nevin S. Scrimshaw

It is a unique privilege for me to share this topic of "Lessons Learned in Controlling the Burden of Malnutrition" with José Maria Bengoa and Igor de Garine. We have seen enormous change in nutrition knowledge and perceptions and in awareness of the importance of nutrition.

We have seen a wide range of nutrition intervention programs, a few successful, some failures, and most somewhere in between. We have seen nutrition permeate almost every field of medicine and public health and have seen recognition of the importance of nutrition to the effectiveness of education, to sound agricultural policies, to the acceptance of family planning, and to measures to lessen the impact and even the prevalence of infectious diseases.

We have had considerable success in iodating salt to prevent the permanent cognitive damage associated with iodine deficiency in pregnancy, and more and more countries are adopting universal fortification of cereal flours with vitamins and minerals.

But we have not seen the end of malnutrition as a scourge of developing countries, and we have not prevented the growing epidemic of nutrition-related chronic disease in nearly all countries.

Unfortunately, overweight and obesity are an even more serious health risk for individuals in these countries, because susceptibility to chronic disease is increased in overweight persons who were undernourished in utero and early childhood. Unfortunately, while the knowledge of human nutrition has progressed rapidly, the programmatic application of this knowledge has fallen far behind. How else to explain the continued high prevalence throughout the developing world of low-birthweight babies, the almost unchecked permanent cognitive damage of iron deficiency in infancy, and the limited impact of programs to reduce the continued stunting of young children in poor populations?

Improved nutrition is absolutely essential to the achievement of nearly all of the UN Millennium Goals, but this is not at all explicit in their presentation. Moreover, the budget and influence of the nutrition programs in the World Health Organization (WHO) and the Food and Agriculture Organization (FAO) have been decreasing.

I believe that the responsibility for the limited success of most public health nutrition programs lies largely with the nutrition community and its priorities. Our nutrition journals are prospering and filled with interesting and relevant research papers. Good nutrition scientists in growing numbers are producing increasingly sophisticated and prestigious research. Nevertheless, even more support is needed for nutrition research and advanced nutrition training, particularly for students from developing countries.

Unfortunately, with some notable exceptions, few of these often brilliant researchers have helped in developing and promoting sound public nutrition policies. In fact, they have often been counterproductive because they lack a preventive and public health perspective and tend to overstress the often-conflicting individual research findings.

Nutrition policy and planning are neglected subjects in academia, even in schools of public health, and can be taught effectively only by persons who themselves have had training and field experience in the formulation and implementation of nutrition and health programs.

Allan Berg's call more than 25 years ago for "nutrition engineers" met with little positive response, perhaps because of resistance to the name. But whatever individuals who can promote nutrition policies and guide interventions are called, public health nutrition does need a large and strong cadre skilled in marshaling science-based nutrition knowledge and applying it effectively to intervention programs. These individuals, working with governments, international agencies, and nongovernmental organizations (NGOs), are an essential complement to talented nutrition researchers. Sometimes a single person is able to fill both roles.

Successful implementation of nutrition policy requires a clear, understandable, and science-based message derived from the best international consensus available. It must not be swayed back and forth by individual researchers interpreting or overvaluing their own limited data. This practice is currently doing great harm to the effectiveness and credibility of public health nutrition efforts, and we must develop more effective consensus mechanisms for limiting the damage this is causing. The traditional role of WHO in providing consensus recommendations on critical nutrition issues should be appreciated and strongly supported, but its response time is often too slow for the pace of modern communication and needs.

The main subjects of this lecture were to be successes, partial successes, and failures. However, as I began to write it, I realized that in good conscience I could not describe any nutrition program as being as successful as global immunization programs leading to the eradication of smallpox, the near eradication of polio, and the sharp decreases in neonatal tetanus, measles, and whooping cough in many if not all countries, or oral rehydration treatment to reduce deaths from diarrhea due to cholera and other causes.

Most of the nutritional successes of the 19th and 20th centuries were not achieved by nutritionists. The striking reductions in mortality from the common communicable disease of childhood, as well as diphtheria, tuberculosis, and pneumonia, came before there were any vaccines or specific therapies for them. Thomas McKeown, in his 1976 book *The Modern Rise of Population*, concludes that the only possible explanation is improved nutrition associated with rising living standards. The same is true for the disappearance as public health problems of the classic nutritional diseases of scurvy, beriberi, pellagra, rickets, kwashiorkor, and keratomalacia.

Obviously public health nutritionists today cannot depend on rising living standards to eliminate the crippling subclinical micronutrient deficiencies damaging the potential of a third of humanity. Moreover, it is now the increase in living standards that is fueling the global epidemic of overweight and obesity with their adverse health consequences.

I am sure that this Congress is only the first of a long series that will strengthen the discipline of public health nutrition, attract

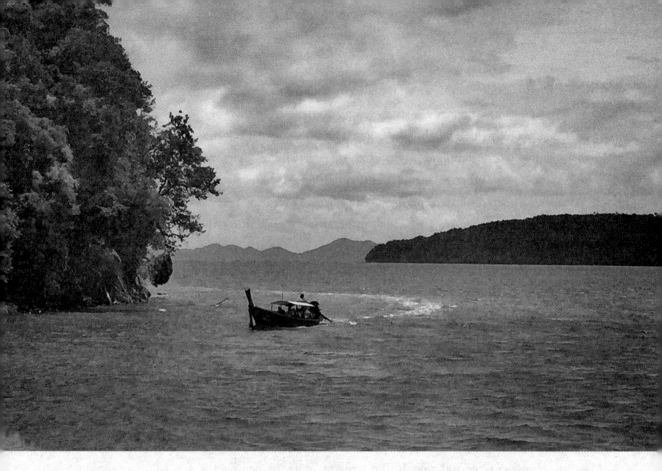

talented professionals to the field，encourage academic programs to train activists in nutrition policy formation and implementation. I hope that it will also help to ensure that the implications of nutrition research findings are understood and communicated from a public health perspective and supported by timely and authoritative expert consensus mechanisms.

(993 words)

※ The text is extracted from the keynote address from the First World Congress on Public Health Nutrition. The author is President of the International Nutrition Foundation, Boston, Massachusetts, USA, and Senior Advisor, United Nations University.

Part Ⅲ Oral Practice

Practice 1
Clinical Inquiry—Department of Cardiology

 Vocabulary

atrial fibrillation	[ˈeɪtrɪəlˌfaɪbrɪˈleɪʃən]	房性纤颤 fibrillation of the muscles of the atria of the heart
cardiac output	[ˈkɑːdiˌæk ˈaʊtpʊt]	心排血量 the amount of blood pumped out by theventricles in a given period of time
cardiac failure	[ˈkɑːdiˌæk ˈfeɪljə]	心力衰竭
oedema	[ɪˈdiːmə]	*n.* (*pl.* oedemata) 水肿；瘤腺体 swelling from excessive accumulation of serous fluid in tissue
dyspnoea	[dɪsˈpniːə]	*n.* 呼吸困难 difficult or labored respiration
arrhythmia	[əˈrɪθmɪə]	*n.* 心律失常,心律不齐 an abnormal rate of muscle contractions in the heart
orthopnoea	[əθɒpˈnɪəə]	*n.* 端坐呼吸 shortness of breath (dyspnea) that occurs when lying flat，causing the person to have to sleep propped up in bed or sitting in a chair
palpitation	[ˌpælpɪˈteɪʃən]	*n.* (*pl.* palpitations)心悸 a rapid and irregular heart beat; a shaky motion
premature beats		房性早搏
multifocal premature ventricular beats		多源性室性早搏
refractory premature ventricular beats		顽固性室性早搏

 Using Lay Terms in Explanations

Explanations should be given in words the patients can understand. Medical terms must be avoided on purpose. Using lay terms—words familiar to people without medical knowledge—can help patients understand explanations. e. g. :

Medical Terms	Lay Terms
1. Dyspnoea	breathlessness/shortness of breath
2. Arrhythmia	palpitations
3. Orthopnoea	breathlessness when lying flat
4. Oedema	swelling

Sample Dialogue

(complaints, medical examination, explanation, advice)

Patient: I get terribly short of breath climbing stairs.

Doctor: How long have you had them?

Patient: I've been getting palpitations.

Patient: For about six months. But I've had heart problems for years, with a long history of heart problems, with tiredness and shortness of breath. In the end I couldn't walk more than a hundred metres without having to stop. I have been increasingly tired, with shortness of breath on exertion, orthopnoea, and palpitatins.

Doctor: (After Examinations) Your pulse is variable between 100 and 180 and was irregular in time. Your blood pressure is 130/80.

Patient: What is the problem?

Doctor: I'll make you an appointment with the electrocardiographic room to have a test. (Or: I'm going to start you on medication to … /I'm going to have you admitted to …)

Doctor: I'm going to have you admitted to the coronary care unit right away so that your treatment can start at once. You'll be given drugs to ease the pain and I expect you'll have an angiogram. They may advise surgery or angioplasty—that's a way of opening up the blood vessels so they can provide more oxygen.

Doctor: There are two suggestions. First, avoid any mental stress and have a good rest. Second, examinations of fasting sugar and an EKG should be done regularly even after the treatment.

Patient: Is it serious?

Doctor: Shortness of breath, or breathlessness, is dyspnoea. At first this is caused by exertion—physical activity such as climbing stairs—but in severe cases it may be present even at rest. A patient who is breathless when lying flat (orthopnoea), for example in bed, will tend to sleep on raised-up two or more pillows. The abbreviation SOBOE stands for shortness of breath on exercise (or on exertion, or on effort).

The normal resting heart rate is 65 – 75 beats per minute. In athletes it may

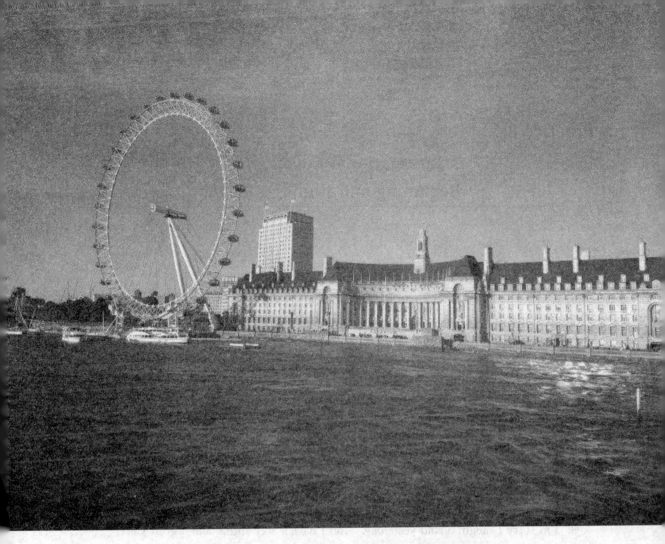

be as low as 40 beats per minute. In extreme athletic activity, the heart rate can go as high as 200/min. The heart rhythm may be regular or irregular. In an irregular rhythm (arrhythmia), there may be early beats which interrupt the regular rhythm (premature beats); or the rhythm may vary with respiration; or it may be completely irregular, as in fibrillation. When patients are aware of irregularity, they describe the symptom as palpitations. Heart failure occurs when the heart is unable to maintain sufficient cardiac output—the amount of blood pumped by the heart each minute—for the body's needs. It may involve the left side of the heart, the right side, or both. In left heart failure the main symptom is breathlessness. The symptoms of right heart failure include peripheral oedema (swelling), beginning in the feet and ankles. This is known as pitting oedema if, when a finger pushed into the swelling, it causes a small depression or pit.

Activities and Role-play (inviting students to improvise and act it out)

Practice 2

International Conference
—Beginning and Ending a Speech

 Useful Expressions for Beginning a Speech

1. I'm particularly honored to have the chance to address you here.
2. It's my great pleasure indeed to be able to read my research paper at this convention.
3. It's a great pleasure to be making my speech about how to slow the aging process, which has been everybody's dream.
4. It's an honor to be invited to make a keynote speech here.
5. The topic today is … . But before that, let me tell you a little about myself.
6. Thank you very much for coming to listen to me despite the bad weather.
7. I hope my speech will be as resourceful, informative as the previous ones.
8. I wish I could draw more attention to my field of study as a result of this speech today.
9. I'm sorry I caught a cold yesterday. And I have a sore throat and a gruff voice.
10. The microphone is in bad shape, so it should be hard to hear me.
11. Does everyone have the handout for my presentation?
12. The most difficult aspect about infant psychology is outlined in the handout.
13. Today I would like to talk about the important problems in the field of abnormal psychology.
14. Today I would like to provide a brief overview of the major findings in my area.
15. Today I will present my view about …

 Useful Expressions for Closing a Speech

1. Our area of study is relatively unknown, so you may hear many unfamiliar phrases in my presentation. I'd like to take a brief moment and let you ask about them.
2. I'd like to spend the last ten minutes on a Q&A session.
3. I would like to leave this question open for my future presentation.
4. Before closing my speech, I would like to point out a problem left for future studies.
5. At the very end of my presentation, let me say a few words of my thanks to the

医学英语学术交流教程

people who gave me valuable suggestions in organizing my presentation.

6. I would like to conclude my presentation. Thank you for your kind attention.

Activities and Role-play (inviting students to improvise and act it out)

Practice 3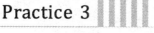

Oral English for Culture and on Social Occasions
—Conference Enrollment

 Occasion: Conference Enrollment

Useful Expressions for Conference Enrollment	
conference registration 会议报名	announcement 会议通知
program 会议日程	arrival information 会议报到
contact 联系方式	speaker 报告人
committee 组委会	

1. Those who haven't paid admission yet, come to pay here, please.
2. This is the desk where you can pay an annual membership fee for this year.
3. Those who haven't paid a fee for the admission, please come up to this desk.
4. There is no need for you to pay the membership fee here.
5. What is the admission, please? /How much do I have to pay for admission?
6. I won't attend the social gathering after the presentation program.
7. What is the total admission?
8. I will only attend the morning session. Would you tell me what the admission is in that case?
9. I'm a new member here. I would like to pay the membership fee.
10. What is the admission fee?

Activities and Role-play (inviting students to improvise and act it out)

Useful Expressions for Dining

Dining places

buffet dinner 自助餐	cafeteria 自助餐厅	banquet hall 宴会厅
revolving restaurant 旋转餐厅	bar 酒吧	snack bar 快餐厅
coffee shop/café 咖啡馆		

Tastes

sour 酸	sweet 甜	bitter 苦
hot/spicy/peppery 辣	salty 咸	

Ways of cooking

fry 煎	stir-fry 炒	deep-fry 炸
steam 蒸	stew 炖	bake 烘烤/焙
roast 炙烤	toast 烤热	

Sauces and Staple Food

Soya sauce 酱油	vinegar 醋	garlic 蒜
black pepper 胡椒	green pepper 青椒	dressings 沙拉调味酱
porridge 稀饭	steamed bread 馒头	steamed rice 蒸米饭
beans 豆	salted vegetables 咸菜	pickled vegetables 泡菜
fried noodles 炒面	rice dumplings wrapped in bamboo leaves 粽子	
deep-fried dough sticks 油条	dumplings 馄饨	bean curd 豆腐
stuffed steamed bun 包子	dumplings 元宵	meat 肉
fish 鱼		

Tableware

coffee pot 咖啡壶	coffee cup 咖啡杯	paper towel 纸巾
napkin 餐巾	table cloth 桌布	tea-pot 茶壶
tea set 茶具	tea tray 茶盘	caddy 茶叶罐
dish 碟子	plate 盘子	saucer 小碟子
bowl 碗	chopsticks 筷子	soup spoon 汤匙
knife 餐刀	cup 杯子	glass 玻璃杯
mug 马克杯	picnic lunch 便当	fruit plate 水果盘
toothpick 牙签		

Sample Sentences

There is a table for four over there.

Would you like to sit over there near the window?

Would you like to order now?

Are you ready to order?

Would you care for a drink/tea/coffee before you order?

How would you like your tea, weak or strong/coffee, black or white?

Do you want anything to start with?

How would you like your steak, rare, medium, or well-down?

Help yourself to the chicken ...

Would you like some more chicken?

Do you want some more chicken?

Would you like some more chicken to eat?

Have some chicken, please.

Many of my fellows are heavy drinkers/in favor of ...

Morning tea needs no order. They will push a trolley over every few minutes, with different sorts of snacks on it each time. You may pick up your favorites.

It makes my mouth water.

I can't help licking my lips.

Would you like to have a second pot/cup?

Topics for Further Discussion

1. Cultural difference between Chinese and American diets
2. Different styles of Chinese cuisines and restaurants
3. Being on diet

References for Further Discussion

1. Eating is one of the key elements in Chinese culture.

Through Chinese food you can taste the greatest Chinese culture. Eating dumplings has been a long tradition for Chinese people. When the Spring Festival comes, every family, rich or poor, makes dumplings. Dumplings are delicious, and we can stuff different things into them to have different flavors. Their shape resembles that of gold ingots（元宝）, a treasured metal currency used in ancient China, symbolizing good fortune.

Chinese people eat noodles very often too, especially on birthdays. It is symbolic of longevity for noodles are long. We have them as a pray for a long life.

Eating is a dominant aspect of the Chinese culture. In China, to have a big feast is one of the most common ways to treat guests. Similar to westerners drinking in a bar with friends, eating together in China is a way to socialize and deepen friendship.

There are many differences between Chinese and American eating habits. One is that unlike in western countries where everyone has his own plate of food, in China, the dishes are placed on the table and everybody shares. As to the amount of food prepared, Americans usually prepare enough food for their guests. However, if you are to be treated by a Chinese host, be prepared for a ton of food. Besides, when eating out together, Americans tend to order their own dishes and often go Dutch, while for a group of Chinese, it is likely that one of them will order for all of them. At the end of the dinner, they will "compete" or even "fight" to pay the bill to show their generosity.

2. The most influential and representative cuisines in China are: Shandong, Sichuan, Guangdong, Fujian, Hunan, Jiangsu, Zhejiang, Anhui cuisines, which are often called Chinese "Eight Cuisines". Each of them can be represented by several exquisite local dishes.

Among all these "Eight Cuisines", Sichuan Cuisine is currently the most popular, best represented by hotpot. Hotpot restaurants are so popular that you can find lovers, families, and groups of friends dining from the same pot, all red-faces and wet-haired. People love it so much that they enjoy it in summer. Yuanyang hotpot is one of the favorite kinds of hotpots. It is so named because half of pot is peppery while the other half is not, looking like the Chinese Yin-yang Diagram. Yuanyang means a couple of lucky birds being loyal to each other all their life-time. Lovers and couples love it for the name.

Foreign-style restaurants are springing up in China like mushrooms in recent years. Japanese sushi, Korean BBQ, Indian curry chicken, McDonald's, KFC, Italian pizza, and Mexican Taco, etc., have become familiar to common Chinese people.

3. Today, there are more and more people going on diet. It keeps people from growing too fat and saves them from many inconveniences and diseases related to being overweight. At the same time, it provides people with sufficient nutrition to keep them in a fit condition. Besides its good effects on people's health, going on a diet can also help many young girls become slim and be able to look good in the latest fashions.

However, if carried too far, going on a diet could become extremely dangerous. Some young girls risk their lives to lose weight because they are eager to have a beautiful figure. The risk can damage their health and even can be life-threatening.

On the whole, being on diet has its positive effects, which also has its side-effects. The proper way of being on diet is to value your health most. If it is good for your health, stick to it; if not, just give it up.

Unit 2

Key Points

Learning Targets

- To master the skill of *listening for the gist*
- To learn the skill of *searching for the main idea*
- To learn about the academic terms of gastroenterology in clinical diagnostic conversation

Learning Focus

- How to raise and answer questions at an international academic conference
- How to pick up guests at airports and help them check in/out at hotels

Cultural Points

- Traditional Chinese medicine

✓音、视频资源
✓参考译文
✓参考答案
✓学术探讨

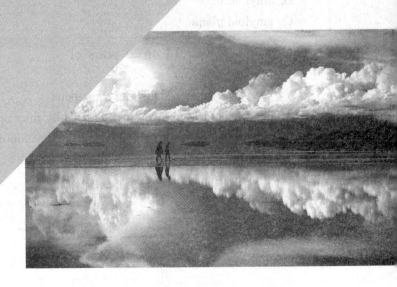

Part I Listening Comprehension

Video 1 ‖‖‖
How to Prevent Alzheimer Disease?

Exercise I Complete the notes below. Write no more than three words in each blank.

The __1__ is where neurotransmitters are released. This is where signals are transmitted, where communication happens. This is where we think, feel, see, hear, __2__ and remember. While the __3__ of Alzheimer's are still debated, most neuroscientists believe that the disease begins when amyloid beta begins to accumulate. And when this happens, it binds to itself, forming sticky aggregates called amyloid plaques. Before it reaches __4__, then triggering a molecular cascade that causes the clinical __5__ of the disease.

Exercise II Write the correct letter A, B, and C in the questions 6—9.

A. synapse
B. amyloid beta
C. amyloid plaque

6. It takes at least 15 or 20 years of _____ accumulation, before it reaches a tipping point.

7. _____ is where Alzheimer's happens.

8. _____ is cleared away metabolized by microglia, the janitor cells of our brains.

9. Drug discovery is largely focused on developing a compound that will prevent, eliminate, or reduce _____ accumulation.

Speech at the 8th International Conference
on Head and Neck Cancer

Exercise Ⅰ Answer the following questions.

1. According to the president's introduction, why was the Milton Dance Head and Neck Center at GBMC established?
2. Which parts are the Dance Center comprised of?
3. Why does Dr. Joseph call Dr. Fu-chan Wei a truly giant in his field?
4. To which field did Dr. Fu-chan Wei make very similar contribution?
5. How does Dr. Fu-chan Wei intentionally entitle his talk?
6. In what cases, can the non-vascularized bone graft not work?

Exercise Ⅱ Listen to the speech and decide whether the following statements are true (T) or false (F).

7. Fu-chan Wei became the chairman of plastic reconstruction surgery in Baltimore.
8. Dr. Fu-chan Wei optimized the functional and esthetic results in order to meet his own taste.
9. Most of techniques may not be useful, especially when there are massive bone defects.
10. Usually there are multiple attempts for reconstruction of the segmental defect.

Listening 1 ▐▐▐▐
Learn to Raise Questions (1)

Exercise Ⅰ Listen to the speech and decide whether the following statements are true (T) or false (F).

1. The first person asking questions is a pediatrician.
2. According to the first person asking questions, children didn't get reported, because children turned out to be insignificant in some way that mattered, but the

efforts were only reports of positive results.

3. In the speaker's opinion, the main reason of children being not included is that they are insignificant.

4. Sarah said the data where we described who was included or not, included only information from the descriptive section of the paper.

5. According to the second person asking questions, most people would not do an analysis by age, because studies are powered for the average treatment effect, and not for age-specific effects.

6. The neonates are less than one month.

7. The speaker believes it is possible to know in the grant proposals if they proposed to do an analysis by age.

8. For the speaker, the question raised by the last person is really a question for the working groups.

Listening 2
Learn to Raise Questions (2)

Exercise Ⅰ Take notes while listening to the audio, and then answer the following questions.

1. How many people raised questions?
2. What are the questions raised?
3. Why do we end up excluding those who are characterized as vulnerable, and pushing potential investigation into their diseases or problems or issues out of the possibility in the research?
4. What's the speaker's opinion upon the question raised by the first person?
5. What's the speaker's answer to the question raised by the second person?

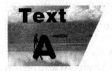
Text A

Comparison between Traditional Chinese Medicine (TCM) and Western Medicine in the Treatment of Diabetes

Kanyeki Ruth Wanjiku

When evaluating patients with diabetes TCM practitioners take a detailed multisystem case history and supplement this information with observations that give information about the state of the patients' health. These observations include: the shape, color and coating of the tongue; the color and expression of the face; the odor of breath and body; the strength, rhythm and quality of the pulse. Many practitioners will palpate along meridians to detect points of tenderness that may indicate a blockage in the flow of Qi at that particular point.

This principle is called symptom and syndrome differentiation. According to western medicine however this concept is not considered but rather only a historical background of the patient is required as well as observing the major symptoms such as checking the heart rate using a stethoscope, checking the blood pressure using the blood pressure monitor or testing the patients urine to check for abnormal insulin levels in the urine.

Unlike western medicine TCM is not concerned with measuring and monitoring blood glucose levels in diabetic patients. Treatment is individualized and geared toward accessing and treating the symptoms that compose patterns of deficiency and disharmony.

Acupuncture and Moxibustion in TCM have been used in the treatment of diabetes to reduce blood insulin levels and normalize the endocrine function. Clinical and experimental studies have demonstrated that acupuncture has a beneficial effect in lowering serum glucose levels. These two methods are beginning to be incorporated into the western forms of treatment although some hospitals do not capitalize on this method as there are not too many doctors who have studied the art.

Both TCM and western medicine share the diabetic treatment goals of reducing symptoms and preventing complications. Both therapies do this by a combination of diet modification, insulin and/or oral pharmacological agents, weight loss where appropriate and regular exercise.

TCM uses a therapy called Percutaneous Nerve Stimulation (PENS) which is a modern adaptation of acupuncture that uses percutaneously placed acupuncture needles to stimulate peripheral sensory and motor nerves innervating pain, the treatment improves physical activity levels, sense of well-being and quality of sleep and reduces oral non-opiodic analgesic medication requirements. The western approach is different as it encourages the use of sleeping pills in case of difficulty in sleeping or use of analgesics prescribed by the doctor.

Herbal prescriptions used in TCM for treating diabetes are formulated or prescribed based on the patients' predominant symptoms. For instance, a patient presenting primarily with excessive thirst i. e. Lung Yin deficiency might be given a single herb such as radix panacis quinquefoli; or a combination of herbs in a patent formulation such as Yu Chuan Wan, which is used in general to treat diabetes of mild to moderate severity. In western medicine the treatment is not individualized but rather a standard prescription is applied to all patients aiming at reducing the blood glucose levels.

TCM herbs must be used with extra caution. Although many formulations have been used safely for centuries in the hands of many trained TCM practitioners, it is important to recognize that data on drug-herb interactions are scarce, and there are clear contraindications to the use of specific herbs in certain populations, such as pregnant women. The prescriptions that are given in western medicine are standard and fixed and hence are safe to be used by patients but also thepatient needs to be keen on the dose prescribed and the time allocated to him or her for consumption of the drug.

TCM and western medicine both incorporate Diet Therapy. This plays an important role in maintaining health and treating disease. In TCM paradigm, foods are valued and prescribed for their energetic and therapeutic purposes rather than solely for their

医学英语学术交流教程

chemical makeup. Western doctors also emphasize on foods with high nutrient levels coked in little or no amount of fats. Attention is paid to the quantity, quality, method of preparation and time of food intake as well as patients' body type, age, vitality, geographical location, and seasonal influences.

TCM uses a concept termed as Qigong which is translated as a function of Qi. It is a meditative method that consists of breathing techniques that can be combined with body movements used as a means in promoting health, healing, spiritual growth and overall well-being. Although it is not a major treatment modality for diabetes, it has been found to be a valuable adjunctive therapy for this condition. Western doctors do not use this concept to improve the patients' well-being but rather advice the patient to keep away from strenuous activities or activities that may strip away the patients peace and sound mind.

TCM uses another concept called Tuina which is a form of Chinese massage that uses hand manipulations such as pulling, kneading, pushing and grasping to stimulate acupuncture points and other parts of the body to create balance and harmony in the system. It can be used effectively in lieu of acupuncture in patients who have an aversion to needles, particularly pediatric patients. This method is not used in western hospitals, and the doctors advise their patients to stretch during exercise as this relaxes and flexes the muscles thus stimulating smooth and regular flow of blood.

Some traditional herbs and prescriptions used for treating diabetes are known to have toxic effects especially if used wrongly or prescribed poorly. The drugs used in western medicine only become toxic if the patient combines the drugs with other medicine that the doctor did not prescribe or overdoses on the prescribed drugs.

In western medicine, the practitioner prescribes hypoglycemic tablets and insulin injection in order to lower the blood glucose level. But this does not address the fact the islets of Langerhans which is responsible for the secretion of insulin is dysfunctional, so when the drug is withdrawn, the blood sugar will rise again. TCM emphasis is not on insulin levels but to create a balance and harmony on the body organs. Hence the herbs used in prescription are used to bring a harmony of all organs thus production of insulin at proper levels.

(1027 words)

Vocabulary

diabetes	[ˌdaɪəˈbiːtiːz]	n. 糖尿病；多尿症
palpate	[pælˈpeɪt]	adj. 有触须的 vt. 触诊
meridian	[məˈrɪdɪən]	n. 经络
stethoscope	[ˈsteθəskəʊp]	n. [临床]听诊器
urine	[ˈjʊərən]	n. 尿
insulin	[ˈɪnsjʊlɪn]	n. [生化][药]胰岛素
pharmacological	[ˌfɑːməkəˈlɒdʒɪkəl]	adj. 药理学的
analgesic	[ˌæn(ə)lˈdʒiːzɪk]	n. 止痛剂；[药]镇痛剂 adj. 止痛的
contraindication	[ˌkɒntrəˌɪndɪˈkeɪʃən]	n. [医]禁忌症
therapeutic	[ˌθerəˈpjuːtɪk]	adj. 治疗的；有益于健康的 n. 治疗剂；治疗学家
meditative	[ˈmedɪˌtətɪv]	adj. 冥想的，沉思的
glucose	[ˈɡluːkəʊs]	n. 葡萄糖
deficiency	[dɪˈfɪʃ(ə)nsɪ]	n. 缺陷，缺点；缺乏
acupuncture	[ˈækjʊˌpʌŋ(k)tʃə]	n. 针刺；[中医]针刺疗法
moxibustion	[ˌmɒksɪˈbʌstʃ(ə)n]	n. 艾灸
endocrine	[ˈendə(ʊ)kraɪn]	n. 内分泌；激素 adj. 内分泌的；激素的
complication	[ˌkɒmplɪˈkeɪʃ(ə)n]	n. 并发症；复杂；复杂化；混乱

◆ **Questions**

1. What are the functions of using Percutaneous Nerve Stimulation?

2. Do you think TCM is less individualized compared to Western medicine? Can you find some evidence from the text?

3. Why should the patients use herbs cautiously? What should patients take into consideration about the prescriptions of Western medicine?

4. Do you think *Qigong* is a major treatment modality for diabetes? Why *Qigong* is used in TCM?

5. In Western medicine, when the drug is withdrawn, why will the blood sugar rise again?

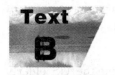

Evaluating Risk of Babesia Infection in the United States, Using CMS and CDC Data Mikhail Menis

Pharm D, MS Epidemiologists, OBE, CBER, FDA

Our presentation is on evaluation of risk of Babesia infection in the United States using CMS and CDC data.

The goal of our evaluation was to establish a database to support benefit-risk analysis for Babesia donor testing. The objectives were to assess babesiosis occurrence among the elderly in the United States using CMS databases, as well as to evaluate babesiosis occurrence in the general population using CDC data, and then to compare babesiosis occurrence overall and by states using CMS and CDC data.

The key point of this analysis is that it substantiates the use of CMS databases for the benefit-risk analysis of Babesia donor screening strategies.

We utilized CMS databases and CDC data to assess occurrence of babesiosis in the United States. Specifically, we used CMS administrative data for calendar years 2006 through 2013 to ascertain incident babesiosis cases, based on the first recording of babesiosis, without prior history of babesiosis diagnosis in the preceding year. Babesiosis occurrence rates per 100,000 US elderly were ascertained overall and by calendar year, diagnosis month, and state of residence. We also used CDC data for 2011 through 2013 to assess babesiosis occurrence rates per 100, 000 residents utilizing US Census data. Then we compared ranking of states for CDC and CMS data, based on babesiosis rates.

The next couple of slides will be on CMS data results. Overall, during the eight-year period, CMS data investigation identified 10,301 unique US elderly medicare beneficiaries with a recorded babesiosis diagnosis and a national babesiosis rate of about 5 per 100,000 elderly Medicare beneficiaries, with state-specific rates up to 10 times higher than the national rate, with significantly increasing babesiosis occurrence in the United States during the eight-year period and the highest rate in 2013, again with the highest babesiosis rates in June, July, and August. Seventy-nine percent of all cases were diagnosed from April through October, similar to the CDC results.

This figure shows babesiosis occurrence among the US elderly by county of residence. As you can see, virtually all the states nationwide except for Wyoming had babesiosis recorded in the elderly, with a substantial concentration of cases occurring in the Northeast corridor, specifically in the top five endemic states.

You can see here in this figure babesiosis cases, the gray bars, and rates, black line, by year among the US elderly Medicare beneficiaries during the eight-year period. As you can see, from 2006 through 2013, babesiosis occurrence is increasing, with the largest number of cases and rate in 2013.

This figure shows babesiosis cases and rates by month of diagnosis among the US elderly medicare beneficiaries during the eight-year period, with the largest number of cases in June, July, and August, and the smallest number of cases in January, February, and March. Again, trends are similar to the CDC data.

Table 1 shows babesiosis cases and rates among the US elderly Medicare beneficiaries overall, by state and year, during the eight-year period. The states are sorted in descending order of babesiosis rate, with the highest rates occurring in the states of Connecticut, Massachusetts, Rhode Island, New York, and New Jersey. Other highlighted states are Babesia-endemic states of New Hampshire, Maine, Minnesota, and Wisconsin.

This slide highlights overall babesiosis cases and rates for the top 15 states, sorted by babesiosis rate on the left in Table 1a and by number of babesiosis cases in Table 1b. As you can see, whether sorted by babesiosis rate or babesiosis cases, the same states end up in both tables, with the highest rates in Connecticut, Massachusetts, Rhode Island, New York, and New Jersey, with the rates per 100,000 in parentheses.

These top five states—Connecticut, Massachusetts, Rhode Island, New York, and New Jersey—accounted for 76. 6 percent of all cases identified in the US elderly. The nine endemic states, including the top five states plus Minnesota, Wisconsin, New Hampshire, and Maine, accounted for 80. 2 percent of all cases in elderly. Other states, as you saw, also had babesiosis recorded, including but not limited to Maryland, Virginia, Pennsylvania,

Florida, and California. The top 15 states, from Connecticut to Florida, by descending babesiosis rate, accounted for 92. 6 percent of all cases. The majority of those 15 states also have significant trends over time. The next slides will be about presenting CDC data on babesiosis occurrence. This Figure 4 shows state-level distribution of babesiosis cases as reported to CDC during 2011 through 2013. As you can see, babesiosis was not reportable in 19 states during the whole period, those states highlighted in gray. They include Pennsylvania, Virginia, and Florida, which do have a substantial number of cases based on CMS data.

Figure 5 shows number of reported cases by year using CDC 2011 through 2013 data, with the highest number of cases occurring in 2013, similar to CMS data. Figure 6 shows number of babesiosis cases by month of symptom onset, CDC 2013 data. Similarly, the largest number of cases occurred in June, July, and August.

This Table 2 shows babesiosis cases and rates in reporting states overall and by year using CDC 2011 through 2013 data, with the states sorted in descending order of babesiosis rate, with the highest rates highlighted in yellow. They are the nine endemic states, starting from Rhode Island, Connecticut, Massachusetts, New York, New Jersey, Maine, New Hampshire, and Wisconsin. Again, the ranking is similar to CMS data, based on babesiosis rate.

The next slide pretty much highlights Table 2, with overall babesiosis cases and rates for the top 15 states, sorted by babesiosis rate on the left and sorted by number of babesiosis cases on the right. As you can see, the top nine states are the same, the endemic states of Rhode Island, Connecticut, Massachusetts, New York, New Jersey, Maine, New Hampshire, Wisconsin, and Minnesota.

In summary, the highest overall babesiosis occurrence rates using CDC data also occurred in the five Northeastern states of Rhode Island, Connecticut, Massachusetts, New York, and New Jersey. These top five Babesia-endemic states accounted for 85. 2 percent of all cases reported to CDC during 2011 through 2013. The top nine endemic states, including the top five states plus Minnesota, Wisconsin, New Hampshire, and Maine, accounted for 98. 5 percent of all cases reported to CDC. The top 15 states from Rhode Island through Nebraska, by descending babesiosis rate, accounted for 99. 4 percent of all babesiosis cases reported to CDC.

This slide shows a comparison of CMS and CDC estimates of

babesiosis rates and corresponding rankings for the top 15 states. As you can see, rankings are similar, especially for the top Babesia-endemic states. For example, if you take Connecticut, it was ranked number 1 based on CMS data and ranked number 2 based on CDC data. New York was ranked number 4 based on CMS data and number 4 based on CDC data. The same ranking occurred in New Jersey and in New Hampshire, which was ranked number 7 in both. So you can see that the ranking based on babesiosis rate is similar for CMS and CDC data.

However, there is a substantially higher rate of babesiosis occurrence using CMS data as compared to CDC data. The next slide will try to summarize that.

Overall, babesiosis results on rankings of state and on occurrence trends over time and by diagnosis months were similar for CMS and CDC data. However, babesiosis occurrence rates identified using CDC case reporting data in general population were substantially lower as compared to babesiosis occurrence identified by CMS data in the US elderly, which could be due to under-reporting or lack of reporting to CDC and a higher likelihood of under-diagnosing babesiosis in the general population versus elderly since babesiosis is more likely to be asymptomatic in younger individuals as compared to older persons. Therefore, we believe that babesiosis occurrence rates among the US elderly Medicare beneficiaries based on CMS data provide the best available population-based estimate of babesiosis occurrence in US blood donors. As such, it was further used to assess number of TTB units prevented and false-positive units diverted, overall and by state, for different blood donor testing strategies, as will be presented next by Dr. Forshee.

CMS data do have limitations. They include:
» Difficulty in identifying incident versus prevalent cases.
» Possible misdiagnosis or mis-recording babesiosis diagnosis.
» Lack of clinical detail for diagnosis code verification.
» Lack of clinical information to ascertain Babesia species.

Thank you so much. I would like to acknowledge the following FDA and CMS and Acumen participants. Now Dr. Forshee will present.

(1437 words)

※ The text is extracted from the keynote address from the Meeting of: The Blood Products Advisory Committee Open Session May 13, 2015; Mikhail Menis, Phar. D., MS Epidemiologists, OBE, CBER, FDA)

 Vocabulary

Babesia	[bəˈbiːzjə]	n. 巴贝虫
CMS	abbr. Centers for Medicare and Medicaid Services	美国医疗保险和医疗补助服务中心
CDC	abbr. Centers for Disease Control	美国疾病控制中心;美国疾病控制和预防中心;美国疾病控制与预防中心
database	[ˈdeɪtəbeɪse]	n. 数据库,资料库
benefit-risk		n. 效益风险;利弊关系
babesiosis	[ˌbæbɪˈzaɪəsɪs]	n. 巴贝虫病
occurrence	[əˈkʌrəns]	n. 发生;出现;事件
substantiate	[səbˈstænʃɪeɪt]	vt. 证明;证实;使实体化
screening strategy		筛选策略
ascertain	[ˌæsəˈteɪn]	vt. 确定;查明;探知
US Census data		美国人口普查数据
ranking	[ˈræŋkɪŋ]	n. 等级;地位;排名
slide	[slaɪd]	n. 滑动;幻灯片
Medicare	[ˈmedɪkeə(r)]	n. 美国国家老年人医疗保险制度;联邦医疗保险
beneficiary	[ˌbenɪˈfɪʃəri]	n. (金融)受益人,受惠者
the Northeast corridor		美国东北走廊铁路线(位于东北部波士顿—华盛顿城市带的电气化铁路线)
endemic	[enˈdemɪk]	adj. (疾病或问题)地方性的,某些人常有的
parentheses	[pəˈrenθəsiːz]	(pl. parenthesis) n. 圆括号;插入语;插入成分
symptom onset		症状出现
asymptomatic	[ˌeɪsɪmptəˈmætɪk]	adj. 无症状的
TTB	abbr. Transfusion-transmitted babesiosis	输血传播巴贝西虫病
false-positive		n. 假阳性

Proper Nouns

Wyoming	美国怀俄明州
Connecticut	康涅狄格州
Massachusetts	马萨诸塞州
Wisconsin	威斯康星州
Rhode Island	罗德岛州

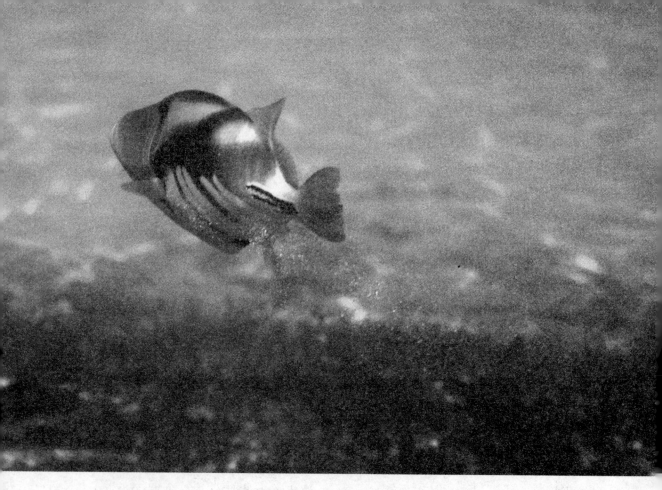

New York	纽约州
New Jersey	新泽西州
New Hampshire	新罕布什尔州
Maine	缅因州
Minnesota	明尼苏达州
Pennsylvania	宾夕法尼亚州
Virginia	弗吉尼亚州
Florida	佛罗里达州
Nebraska	内布拉斯加州

◆ Questions

1. What are the three objectives for this keynote speech?
2. According to CMS data, in which year did babesiosis occurrence reach the highest rate?
3. Were CMS and CDC results similar in babesiosis rates by month of diagnosis?
4. What were the top nine endemic states of the disease and what was the percentage of them based on CDC data?
5. In what ways were CDC data and CMS data different in babesiosis occurrence rates? And why?

医学英语学术交流教程

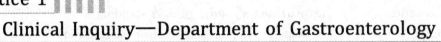

Part III Oral Practice

Practice 1
Clinical Inquiry—Department of Gastroenterology

 Vocabulary

heartburn	['hɑːtbɜːn]	*n.* 胃灼热,烧心 an unpleasant burning feeling in your stomach or chest caused by acid from your stomach
sodium bicarbonate	['səudɪəm][baɪ'kɑːbənɪt]	*n.* 碳酸氢钠;小苏打 a white powder used in baking or for cleaning things
nausea	['nɔːzɪə]	*n.* 恶心,晕船 the feeling that you have when you think you are going to vomit
bowels	['bauəlz]	*n.* 肠 the tubes in your body through which digested food passes from your stomach to your anus
stool	[stuːl]	*n.* 粪便 a piece of solid waste from your bowels
abdomen	['æbdəmən]	*n.* 腹部;腹腔 the part of the body between the chest and pelvis
duodenal	[ˌdjuːəu'diːnəl]	*adj.* 十二指肠的 relating to or contained in the duodenum
ulcer	['ʌlsə]	*n.* 溃疡;腐烂物 a sore area on your skin or inside your body that may bleed or produce poisonous substances
X-ray film		X 射线胶片
gastrointestinal tract	[ˌgæstrəuɪn'testɪn(ə)l]	*n.* 胃肠道 an organ system which takes in food, digests it to extract and absorb energy and nutrients, and expels the remaining waste
duodenum	[ˌdjuːə'diːnəm]	*n.* 十二指肠 the top part of the bowel, below the stomach

indigestion	[ˌɪndɪˈdʒestʃ(ə)n; -daɪ-]	*n.* 消化不良 pain that you get when your stomach cannot break down food that you have eaten
complication	[ˌkɒmplɪˈkeɪʃ(ə)n]	*n.* 并发症 a medical problem that happens while someone is already ill and makes treatment more difficult
melena	[məˈliːnə]	*n.* 黑粪症 the black, tarry feces that are associated with upper gastrointestinal bleeding
orthostatic	[ˌɔːθə(ʊ)ˈstætɪk]	*adj.* 直立的 standing
syncope	[ˈsɪŋkəpɪ]	*n.* 晕厥 faint or passing out
hematemesis	[ˌhiːməˈteməsɪs]	*n.* 吐血;呕血 vomiting of blood
fluids	[ˈfluɪdz]	*n.* 流食 liquid food
tepid	[ˈtepɪd]	*adj.* 微温的,温热的 slightly warm

 Using Lay Terms in Explanations

Explanations should be given in words the patients will understand, avoiding medical terms. Using lay terms—words familiar to people without medical knowledge—can help patients understand explanations. e. g. :

Medical Terms	**Lay Terms**
1. ulcer	a break in the inner lining (of an organ)
2. melena	lack tarry stools
3. orthostatic syncope	passing out upon standing
4. hematemesis	vomiting blood

Sample Dialogue

Patient: I have a pain in my stomach.

Doctor: How long have you had it?

Patient: I have had it off and on (intermittently) for the past three years. It has been really bad these past two weeks.

Doctor: Do you feel it only when your stomach is empty?

Patient: Yes. After I eat, it goes away for a while.

Doctor: When do you get it?

Patient: Usually when I get very nervous. Sometimes it awakes me up in the middle of the night.

Doctor: What kind of pain do you have?

Patient: It gives me a burning sensation, like heartburn.

Doctor: Usually how do you get relief?

Patient: After I take some sodium bicarbonate, the pain goes away temporarily.

Doctor: Have you had any nausea or vomiting?

Patient: Yes, occasionally.

Doctor: Are your bowels regular? Have you observed your stools?

Patient: I usually have to go once every other day. I was very worried because last night I went twice and the color was black.

Doctor: Let me examine your abdomen. Lie down on your back and bend your knees up please.

Doctor: (After examination) It sounds like a duodenal ulcer, but we have to do some tests, and take an X-ray film of your gastrointestinal tract first, before we can be certain.

Patient: Is it serious?

Doctor: A break in the inner lining of the duodenum is called duodenal ulcer. Many ulcer patients experience minimal indigestion, abdominal discomfort that occurs after meals. Some complain of upper abdominal burning or hunger pain one to three hours after meals or in the middle of the night. Others may have a serious complication, like bleeding. Patients with ulcer bleeding may report passage of black tarry stools (melena), weakness, a sense of passing out upon standing (orthostatic syncope), and vomiting blood (hematemesis).

Patient: So what should I do with this disease?

Doctor: You should have a complete rest and give your stomach as little work as possible. Take only fluids. There is nothing better than boiled tepid milk taken regularly in small quantities. In addition, I will give you some medicine. If the black stools persist or your condition gets worse, come back to the hospital at once.

Patient: Thank you so much. I'll follow your advice.

Additional Expressions for Digestive System Diseases

belching 嗳气	sour regurgitation 反酸
diarrhea 腹泻	bloody stool 血便
watery stool 水样便	mucous stool 粘液便
bowel movement 排便	dyspepsia 消化不良
constipation 便秘	abdominal distension 腹胀
appendicitis 阑尾炎	abdominal pain 腹痛
upper abdomen 上腹部	lower abdomen 下腹部
umbilical part/region 脐部	peptic ulcer 消化性溃疡
intestinal obstruction 肠梗阻	acute gastroenteritis 急性肠胃炎

1. How long have you had abdominal pain? Can you show me where it is?

2. Are you vomiting? What do you vomit? What does it look like?

3. How is your appetite?

4. Have you ever taken any contaminated food?

5. How many bowel movements have you had a day?

6. What kind of stool did you notice? Watery or mucous?

7. Is there any bloody stool?

8. Do you have abdominal pain when you have diarrhea?

9. I need a specimen of your stool for test.

10. You must take more fluids, and just have a light diet until you feel better.

Activities and Role-play (inviting students to improvise and act it out)

Practice 2

International Conference
—Raising and Answering a Question

Useful Expressions for Raising a Question

A. Direct Questioning

1. I would like to ask (address/put/raise/pose) a question to Mr. A.

2. Dr. A, may I ask you two questions?

3. I'd like to raise two questions about (regarding/concerning)... and direct them to Prof. A.

4. A question for Dr. A, have you tried this technique?

5. My second question is the following.

6. May I ask Mr. A to tell us how you synthesized the sample?

7. What I'm asking is, did you measure the temperature of the system?

8. What I'd like to ask Prof. A is, is it possible to measure the molecular weight by GC – MS?

9. Could you please tell us what you really mean by evidence-based medicine?

10. Could you provide any example to prove what you have said about immunotherapy?

B. Indirect Questioning

1. Mr. A, I wonder if you would like to comment on this point.

2. I wonder if you would be kind enough to explain/clarify it.

3. What I'm wondering is whether it is possible to measure the parameter by this technique.

4. I am curious, regarding your last slide, why you used this method in your experiments.

5. I am anxious(eager) to hear Mr. A's opinion about precision medicine.

6. I am interested in how you would compare ... with ... .

7. I'd be glad to know if the procedure will help me to synthesize some new compounds.

8. I believe it would be most useful, Dr. A, if you pointed out how this material plays a role in the kinetics.

 ## Useful Expressions for Answering a Question

A. Identifying the Question

1. Are you asking me question about ... ?

2. I'm not quite sure what your question is (what you mean).

3. I didn't quite get the last point of your question.

4. Could you be more specific about your question?

5. I don't know whether I have understood your question correctly. Do you mean ... ?

B. Before Answering the Question

1. That's a good (relevant/important/interesting/difficult/complicated) question.

2. I appreciate that question.

3. Thank you for asking that question.

4. I think your question is really to the point.

5. I'm very glad you asked this question, because ...

C. Giving a Direct Answer

1. I wish (would like) to answer Mr. A's question.

2. Let me first reply very rapidly to the first question.

3. May I answer your second question first?

4. Allow me to respond to that question briefly.

5. In answer to the second question, I would say that ...

6. My answer to that question is that ...

7. I'll try to answer your question by using ... as an example.

8. Let me try to answer these questions one by one.

D. Giving a Partial Answer

1. I can only provide a partial answer to that question.

2. In partial answer to Dr. A's question, it may be relevant to indicate that we are studying ...

3. That is one possible explanation, but it is certainly not the only one.

4. At the present time, I can only express a few highly speculative ideas.

5. As far as I know, no enough study has been made on that area.

E. Giving a Promising Answer

1. The study has not yet progressed to that point. But I hope a year from now I'll be able to show you the data.

2. We are now working on this problem and, if you agree, I will answer your question in a few weeks.

3. I think it will be possible to answer this question when more experiments are completed.

4. The answer to this question is going to need further study.

5. Not at present time. Perhaps later. (abbreviated answer)

F. Facing a Tough Question

1. I(really/honestly) don't know.

2. I'm afraid/sorry I don't know anything about … .

3. I'm not sure I can answer that question.

4. It's difficult to answer that question.

5. What I'm going to say is not quite an answer to the question at this time.

6. I'm afraid I have no idea how to answer your question.

7. I don't have any evidence (data/information) regarding your question.

8. I have had very little experience with this matter.

9. This kind of experiment hasn't been done yet. This certainly is an important experiment for future consideration.

G. After Answering the Question

1. Does that answer your question?

2. Is this what you wanted me to say?

3. I hope this answers your question.

4. I don't know if that is a satisfactory answer.

5. I hope this may serve as an answer to Mr. A.

6. Is that responsive to your question?

 Useful Expressions for Stating Personal Opinion

A. Unemphatic Statements

1. I'd like to make a few comments/remarks to clarify some of the points made earlier that I believe might be misunderstood.

2. I just want to remark on the last point Dr. A made.

3. I'd like to offer (present/give/express/state) my opinion on this subject.

4. In my opinion … is perhaps the most important discovery in medicine.

5. I have an impression/a feeling that this mechanism should be in category A.

6. I am under impression that there is a close relationship between ... and ...

7. What I am trying to say is there is no correlation between ... and ...

8. I think (believe/consider/regard/suppose) that the theory is sound.

9. I feel strongly that the results should be viewed as a great advance in this field.

10. It seems to me that he is hiding some important facts.

B. Emphatic Statements

1. The point is that the effect of the compound may vary as a function of concentration.

2. I'd like to place (put/lay) emphasis on the fact that no drug is absolutely safe.

3. I'd like to focus your attention on ...

4. Let me emphasize (underline/underscore) the limitations of this theory.

5. We have enough reason to believe that man would be sensitive to these stimuli.

6. I'm sure everyone in the audience knows that this polymer is a semi-crystalline material.

7. Let me point out one more thing.

8. I don't think there is need for a formal summary, but I do have a few points to make.

Activities and Role-play (inviting students to improvise and act it out)

Practice 3

Oral English for Culture and on Social Occasions
—Airport Pick-up and Hotel Accommodation

 Occasion: Airport Pick-up

Useful Expressions for Airport Pick-up

information desk 问询处	airport terminal 机场候机楼
flight number (FLT No.) 航班号	scheduled time (SCHED) 预计时间
delay 延误	duty-free shop 免税店
currency exchange 货币兑换处	security checkpoint 安检处
passport control 护照检查处	luggage claim/baggage claim 行李领取处
luggage tag 行李牌	goods to declare 报关物品
ticket office 购票处	taxi pick-up point 出租车乘车点
coach pick-up point 长途客车乘车点	

Sample Sentences for Greeting and Introduction

1. Excuse me, Sir. Are you Prof. Goodman from New York?
2. Hi, I'm Li Ming, director of the Beijing office. I've come to meet you. Here is my name card. Welcome to Beijing.
3. Nice to meet you. And this is my secretary, Miss Wang.
4. Mr. Sun, I'd like you to meet Mr. Johnathan Mitchell, sales manager for Northern Reflections of Canada.
5. It's very nice to finally meet you, Prof. Goodman, after so many emails. I'd like you to have my name card.

Sample Sentences for Guide and Service

1. Do you know where the luggage claim area is?
2. Have you got your luggage?
3. How many pieces of luggage do you have?
4. Let's go this way, please. Our car is over there.
5. Here's the car. Step in, please.
6. We've reserved/booked a room for you in the Green Hotel. Shall we go to the hotel directly?
7. We'll go there by taxi. This way please.
8. If all is ready, we'd better start for the hotel.
9. We hope you could enjoy our arrangement.
10. I wish you a pleasant stay here.
11. There's no arrangement tomorrow. Have a good rest and recover from the jet lag.
12. This is the schedule for tomorrow.
13. If you have any problems on your life or business, please don't hesitate to call me.

Activities and Role-play (inviting students to improvise and act it out)

Occasion：Hotel Accommodation

Useful Expressions for Hotel Accommodation

information counter 服务台	registration 登记处	check in 入住登记
check out 退房离开	book/reserve 预订	vacancy 空房
room charge 房价	special rate 优惠价	discount 折扣
credit card 信用卡	cash 现金	luggage/baggage 行李
suitcase 行李箱	valuable 贵重物品	breakable 易碎的
departure date 离店日期	receipt 收据	fine 罚金
bill 账单	invoice 发票	deposit 押金
off-season 淡季	peak-season 旺季	extension 电话分机
telephone directory 电话号码本		

Type of Room

double room 双人房	single room 单人房	twin room 标准间
suite 套房	deluxe suite 豪华套房	presidential suite 总统套房
with (a) bath 附浴室的	with a balcony 附阳台的	with (a) shower 附淋浴设备的
with kitchen facilities 附厨房设备的	with a good view 视野好的	
with breakfast 附早餐的	with full board 附三餐的	
on the sunny side 向阳的	overlooking the sea 俯瞰海景的	
facing the garden 面向花园的	with air conditioning 附空调设备的	

Sample Dialogue 1：Check-in

Guest： Good evening.

Receptionist：Good evening, Ma'am. May I help you?

Guest： Yes. I'd like to check in, please. I made a reservation a week ago under the name of Ruby Hsu, H—S—U, for three nights from tonight. And here is my confirmation slip.

Receptionist：Thank you, Miss Hsu. A second, please ... Oh, yes, we've got your reservation. It is a single room with bath. Is it correct?

Guest： Yeah, correct.

Receptionist：Then, please fill out this form, Miss Hsu.

Guest： Sure. (Fill out the registration card.) Is this OK?

Receptionist：Thank you. Your room number is 666 and here is your room key. Just leave your baggage here and I'll get the porter to carry it up right away.

Guest： Thank you very much.

Receptionist：My pleasure.

Sample Dialogue 2: Check-out

Guest: Check out, please.

Cashier: Your room number, please?

Guest: Oh, the room number is 666 and here is the key.

Cashier: Thank you. Did you enjoy your stay with us here?

Guest: Very much. The room was comfy and the service was great.

Cashier: Thank you. That's good to hear. Here is your bill. The total is three hundred and forty-five dollars, tax included. How would you like to pay?

Guest: I'll pay by my credit card, but I'll need a receipt so I can charge it to my company.

Cashier: Absolutely. Here we are, sir. If you like you can leave your bags with the porter and he can load them onto the shuttle for you when it arrives.

Guest: That would be great, thank you.

Cashier: Our pleasure. Thank you again for staying at the Woodward Hotel.

Additional Sentences for Hotel Accommodation

1. I'd like a single room with bath and a good view.
2. Do you have a double room overlooking the sea?
3. Excuse me, can I have a wake-up call at seven tomorrow morning?
4. Would you please keep the valuables for me?
5. Would you please bring me up some towels?
6. The room's air-conditioning doesn't work. I want to change my room, but to a room with a view as good as this one.
7. Are there any free drinks in the fridge?
8. What kind of facilities do you have in the hotel?
9. Could I use the swimming pool for free?
10. When does the breakfast finish?
11. Which floor is the restaurant located?
12. Is there any discount if I stay for three nights?

Activities and Role-play (inviting students to improvise and act it out)

Cultural Topics for Further Discussion

1. The basic principles of traditional Chinese medicine
2. Four methods of diagnosis in traditional Chinese medicine
3. Chinese medical herbs
4. Chinese acupuncture and moxibustion

References for Further Discussion

1. China was one of the first countries to have a medical culture. In comparison with Western methods, Chinese medicine takes a far different approach. With a history of 5,000 years, it has formed a deep and immense knowledge of medical science, diagnostic methods, prescriptions and cures. The basic principles are rather distinctive:

Relative Properties—*Yin* and *Yang*

The physiology of Chinese medicine holds that the human body's life is the result of the balance of *yin* and *yang*. *Yin* is the inner and negative principles, and *yang*, outer and positive. The key reason why there is sickness is because the two aspects lose their harmony. Seen from the recovery mechanism of organs, *yang* functions to protect from outer harm, and *yin* is the inner base to store and provide energy for its counterpart.

Basic Substance

Doctors of traditional Chinese medicine (abbreviated to TCM) believe that vital energy—moving and energetic particles, state of blood, and body fluid are the essential substances that compose together to form the human body, and the basis for internal organs to process. They are channeled along a network within the body—*Jingluo* as their channels. On the physical side, vital energy serving to promote and warm belongs to the properties of *yang*, and blood and body fluid to moisten possesses the properties of *yin*.

2. It is a wonder that TCM doctors could cure countless patients without any assistant apparatus but only a physical examination. The four methods of diagnosis consist of observation, auscultation and olfaction, interrogation, pulse taking and palpation.

Observation indicates that doctors directly watch the outward appearance to know a patient's condition. As the exterior and interior correspond immediately, when the inner organs run wrongly, it will be reflected through skin pallor, tongue, the facial sensory organs and some excrement.

Auscultation and olfaction is a way for doctors to collect messages through hearing the sound and smelling the odor. This is another reference for diagnosis.

Interrogation suggests that doctors question the patient and his relatives, so as to know the symptoms, evolution of the disease and previous treatments.

The taking of the pulse and palpation refers that doctors noting the pulse condition of patients on the radial artery, and then to know the inner change of symptom. Doctors believe that when the organic function is normal, the pulse, frequency, and intension of pulse will be relatively stable, and when not, variant.

3. In traditional Chinese medical science, the drugs are also different from the West, because doctors have discovered the medicinal effects of thousands of herbs over a long period of time. Doctors would analyze their nature or property such as "cold and hot" or "*yin* and *yang*", utilize all sorts of raw materials, mixing them to cure disease. Before taking the medicine, the patient will have to boil it. Then there is the distinctive method of preparation, associated with the acupuncture and massage, the treatment will take effect magically.

About the classification, in the *Compendium of Materia Medica* by Li Shizhen in the Ming Dynasty, there are 1892 types recorded, giving the detailed information.

Such a complicated medical science had come down thanks to records like *The Yellow Emperor's Canon of Interior Medicine*, Shen Nong's *Canon of Herbs*, *and the Compendium of Materia Medica*, which are all comprehensive and profound works. There are also wide-spread stories praising the experienced and notable doctors in ancient China like Hua Tuo in the Three Kingdoms Periods. Today, though western medicine has been adopted, traditional treatments are still playing an important role and have raised great attention and interest worldwide due to the amazing curative effects.

4. Acupuncture and massage have become more and more accepted within the medicine field of the world. What fascinates people is that fine needles and the gentle strength can make you healthy without taking lots of pills. Actually it consists of two parts: operations with needles and ones with fire, both of them are essential and correlative during curing.

Operations with Needles

This field features the pricks of needles on acupuncture points (acupoints for short) to adjust the organic functions and clear the energy channels of obstruction in our body.

In ancient China, it was a treat method with stone needles which then evolved into the bone, bamboo, and metal. Now it is popular to use stainless steel and silver needles among the doctors of Chinese medicine.

After thousands of years' clinical practice and summaries, complete theoretical systems came into being. According to the records, it is on the passages named *jingluo* through which vital energy circulates around the whole body. If the passages like a network are blocked, doctors will prick acupoints to dredge them. On the passages, there dispersed hundreds of acupoints. Once the needle enters into the acupoints, deep or shallow, lifted or entwisted, inserted in different frequency, all according to the techniques of experienced doctors, the miraculous effect will appear.

Operations with Fire

In Chinese language from the linguistic angle, the character *jiu* that represents this kind of operations—moxibustion, has a pictographic element of fire, that is to say, this method of treatment must have a close relation with fire.

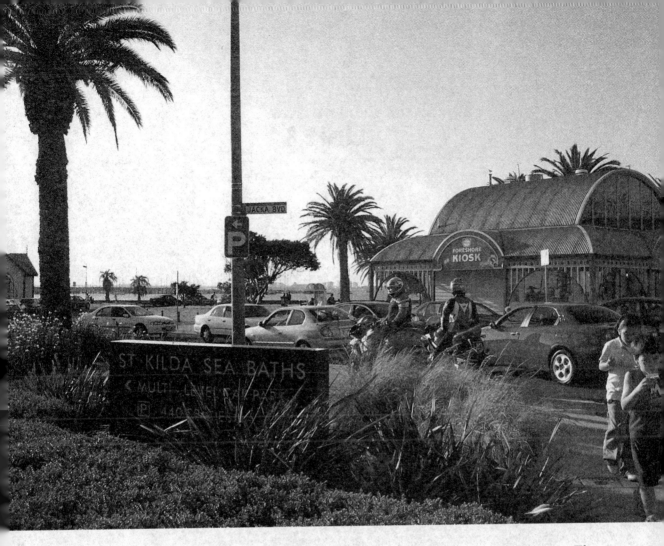

The methods in common use are moxibustion with moxa cone and cupping. The principle of cupping lies in that, when the fire in the jar is burnt, heating power ejects the air out, and the negative pressure makes the jar stick to the skin, which causes the stasis of blood to stimulate and adjust the organ functions, the moxa cone can also have this effect.

Unit 3

Key Points

....

Learning Targets
- To master the skill of *listening for details*
- To learn the skill of *scanning for details*
- To learn about the academic terms of respiratory system in clinical diagnostic conversation

Learning Focus
- How to do discussions and make comments at an international academic conference

Cultural Points
- Chinese scenic spots and historic sites

✓音、视频资源
✓参考译文
✓参考答案
✓学术探讨

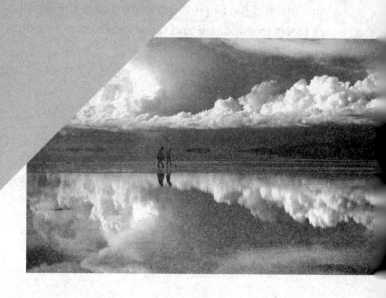

Video 1

The Wireless Future of Medicine

Exercise Ⅰ Choose correct answers to the following questions.

1. When was the stethoscope invented?
   A. 1860　　　　B. 1680　　　　C. 1618　　　　D. 1816
2. In the future, what will be the doctors walking around with to check a patient's vital signs?
   A. a stethoscope　　　　　　　B. a smart phone
   C. a digital camera　　　　　　D. a video player
3. What can't an expectant parent monitor on a smart phone in the future?
   A. fetal heart rate　　　　　　　B. intrauterine contraction
   C. temperature outside mother's body   D. state of amniotic fluid
4. What disease has been impacted by continuous glucose sensors?
   A. cardiac disease   B. diabetes   C. pneumonia   D. hepatitis
5. According to this passage, which can be taken measurement of intake and expenditure by a Band-Aid in the future?
   A. Calcium　　　B. Calorie　　　C. Copper　　　D. Iron

Exercise Ⅱ Decide whether the following statements are true (T) or false (F).

6. A cardiologist can watch a patient's rhythm through a smart phone nowadays.
7. Today we can't check all our vital signs anywhere in the world on our smart phones yet.
8. In the future, continuous glucose sensors needn't be implanted under the skin.
9. In a few years, we can have every minute of our sleep displayed on our smart phones.
10. The Holter Monitor is an obsolete technology now and will be soon buried.

Video 2

One More Reason to Get a Good Night's Sleep

Exercise Ⅰ   Watch the video and then answer the following questions.

1. How much time do we spend sleeping in our lives?

2. What did Galen think of the role of sleep?

3. What's the first problem that every organ must solve?

4. How much energy supply does brain use for its electrical activity?

5. Which system solves the nutrient delivery problem and how?

Exercise Ⅱ   Take notes while watching the video, and then complete the following sentences.

Now, just as every cell requires nutrients to __6__ it, every cell also produces waste as a __7__ , and the clearance of that waste is the second basic problem that each organ has to solve. This diagram shows the body's __8__ system, which has evolved to meet this need. It's a second parallel network of vessels that extends throughout the body. It takes up __9__ and other waste from the spaces between the cells, it collects them, and then dumps them into the blood so they can be __10__ of.

Listening 1

The Potential of Regenerative Medicine

Exercise Ⅰ   Fill in the blanks with the missing words and expressions.

Here's a dolphin where the fin's been __1__ . There are now __2__ patients around the world who have used that material to heal their wounds. Could you regenerate a limb? DARPA just gave Steve 15 million dollars to lead an eight-institution project to begin the process of asking that question.

And I'll show you the 15 million dollar picture. This is a 78 year-old man who's lost __3__. After treatment that's what it looks like. This is happening today. This is __4__ today. There are materials that do this. Here are the heart patches.

But could you go a little further? Could you, say, instead of using material, can I take some cells along with the material, and remove a damaged piece of tissue, put a __5__ material on there? You can see here a little bit of heart muscle beating in a dish. This was done by Teruo Okano at Tokyo Women's Hospital. He can actually grow __6__ in a dish. He chills the dish, it changes its __7__ and he peels it right out of the dish. It's the coolest stuff.

Now I'm going to show you __8__. And what I'm going to show you here is stem cells __9__ the hip of a patient. Again, if you're squeamish, you don't want to watch. But this one's kind of cool. So this is a bypass operation, just like what Al Gore had, with a difference. In this case, at the end of the bypass operation, you're going to see the stem cells from the patient that were removed at the beginning of the procedure __10__ into the heart of the patient. And I'm standing up here because at one point I'm going to show you just how early this technology is. Here go the stem cells, right into the beating heart of the patient. And if you look really carefully, it's going to be right around this point you'll actually see a back-flush. You see the cells coming back out. We need all sorts of new technology, new devices, to get the cells to the right place at the right time.

Exercise II   Decide whether the following statements are true (T) or false (F).

11. When we hear about diabetic ulcers, we naturally think of amputation as the final treatment.
12. The horse healed up after being treated with the new therapy invented by Steve.
13. We can remove the stem cells from one's hip and directly inject them into one's heart with the new technology.
14. No patients with heart diseases can be brought back to an asymptomatic state with the new therapy.
15. The new technology has treated many patients with their own liposuction fluid.

Listening 2
Learn to Raise Questions (3)

Exercise I   Decide whether the following statements are true (T) or false (F).

1. Due to lack of the data, doctors don't know if a treatment for someone who is

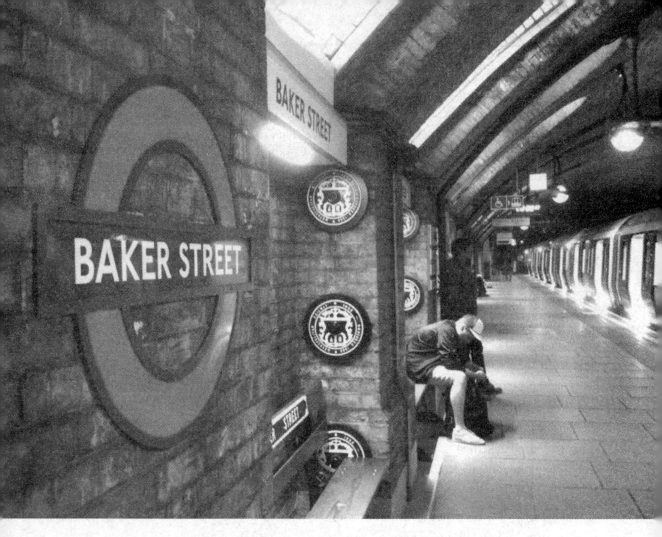

pregnant and/or breast feeding can take the medications that she needs.

2. Doctors have enough information to make an evidence-based decision of whether it's sick women getting pregnant or pregnant women getting sick.

3. The speaker said they had worked with Dr. Bianca to have a conference on enrolling pregnant women in clinical research, and call for the creation of a research agenda around that space.

4. They are care-givers, and geriatrician members who are interested in Alzheimer's disease, so women are willing to participate in trials.

5. There is an increasing number of baby boomers in the sandwich generation, but they don't take care of both children and elderly relatives.

6. Four persons raised questions.

7. The last question raised is about the sex as a biological variable.

8. As for the last question, the speaker said it was a process involving requests for information from the scientific community, a trans-NIH sex by a biological variable working group, a collaboration with the trans-NIH working group and a variety of other consultations.

医学英语学术交流教程

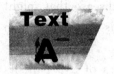

Diabetes and Deafness
—Is It Sufficient to Screen for the Mitochondrial 3243A>G Mutation Alone?

Roger G. Whittaker

The m. 3243A>G mitochondrial DNA mutation is well known to be associated with deafness and diabetes, and patients presenting with these clinical features are routinely screened for this mutation. We wanted to assess whether this is a suitable screening strategy. We retrospectively reviewed the clinical notes of 242 patients who had attended a special mitochondrial clinic in the preceding 25-year period. Of the total 29 patients with mitochondrial disease presenting with deafness and diabetes, only 21 would have been correctly diagnosed by screening for the m. 3243A>G mutation in blood or urine. Of the remaining eight patients, only six had other features suggestive of mitochondrial disease. We recommend that all patients with the combination of deafness and diabetes presenting to diabetes clinics be screened for the m. 3243A>G mutation. In those patients in whom this test is negative, we recommend referral to a specialist neuromuscular clinic for further investigation.

RESEARCH DESIGN AND METHODS—The association between maternally inherited diabetes and deafness and mitochondrial DNA (mtDNA) mutations is well recognized (1, 2). Several mutations have been associated with this phenotype, including the m. 3243A>G (3) and m. 14709T>C (4) point mutations. The association is so strong with the m. 3243A>G mutation (thought to account for up to 1% of diabetes and 0.3% of deafness [5 – 7]) that it has become common practice in diabetes clinics for patients presenting with the combination of diabetes and deafness to be screened for this mutation in either whole-blood or urinary epithelial cells (8). We wanted to assess whether this is a sensible investigation strategy in patients presenting in this way. First, we wanted to assess how many patients with other mutations of the mitochondrial genome present with the combination of diabetes and deafness would potentially be missed in this screening strategy. Second, we wanted to investigate whether other clinical features of mitochondrial disease that might provide additional clues as to the correct diagnosis were present in these patients (9).

We retrospectively reviewed the clinical notes of 242 patients who had attended a specialist mitochondrial clinic in the preceding 25-year period. All patients had proven mitochondrial disease on the basis of muscle histochemistry or mtDNA analysis. From this cohort, we selected patients who were deaf at the time at which they presented with diabetes. Diabetes was defined according to World Health Organization criteria (10). Deafness was clinically defined as hearing impairment not fully corrected with hearing aids. Audiometry was not deemed necessary, as this is unlikely to have been performed at the time of presentation to a diabetes clinic.

RESULTS—We found a total of 29 patients with mitochondrial disease who were deaf at the time of presentation with diabetes. Twenty-one of these patients carried the m. 3243A > G point mutation, with deafness having preceded diabetes by a mean of 6. 0 years. In addition, there were two patients with the m. 12258C>A mutation, one with the m. 8344A>G mutation, four with single large-scale mtDNA deletions, and one with multiple mtDNA deletions secondary to an unknown nuclear genetic defect.

The clinical features of these eight patients who did not carry the m. 3243A>G mutation are summarized in Table 1. The patient with m. 8344A>G also had ptosis, dysarthria, and cerebellar ataxia at the time of presentation with diabetes. One patient with the m. 12258C>A mutation had no other clinical features, whereas the other had only mild constipation, fatigue, and a mild dysarthria. Three of the patients with single mtDNA deletions had clear evidence of mitochondrial disease with ptosis, marked external ophthalmoplegia, and clear dysarthria. However, the fourth had only a history of mild fatigue in addition to deafness and diabetes. The patient with multiple mtDNA deletions also had ptosis and ophthalmoplegia.

Of the total 29 patients with mitochondrial disease presenting with deafness and diabetes, 21 would have been correctly diagnosed with mitochondrial disease by screening for the m. 3243A＞G mutation in blood or urine. The remaining eight patients would not have been detected by this screening strategy, underestimating the prevalence of diabetes and deafness due to mtDNA mutations. Six of these patients had other clear signs of mitochondrial disease. It is likely that these patients would have been referred for a neurological opinion and the correct diagnosis made. However, one patient with the m. 12258C＞A mutation and one with a single deletion had either no other features or only nonspecific features (i. e. fatigue) that are unlikely to have alerted the assessing physician to the possibility of an alternative diagnosis.

CONCLUSIONS—We recommend that all patients presenting to diabetes clinics with the combination of deafness and diabetes be screened for the m. 3243A＞G mutation. Screening of urine is preferred, as this has a greater sensitivity than either buccal mucosa or blood (8 – 11), is noninvasive, and is widely available. However, in those patients in whom this test is negative, we recommend referral to a specialist neuromuscular clinic for further investigation to ensure that patients harboring other mtDNA mutations are correctly diagnosed.

(841words)

※ The text is extracted from *Diabetes Care*, Volume 30, Number 9, September 2007.

 ## Vocabulary

mitochondrial	[ˌmaɪtəʊˈkɒndrɪəl]	*adj.* 线粒体的
mutation	[mjuːˈteɪʃ(ə)n]	*n.* [遗]突变；变化；元音变化
referral	[rɪˈfɜːrə(ə)l]	*n.* 参照；提及；被推举的人；转诊病人
phenotype	[ˈfiːnə(ʊ)taɪp]	*n.* 表型，表现型；显型
urinary epithelial cells		尿路上皮细胞
audiometry	[ˌɔːdɪˈɒmətrɪ]	*n.* [耳鼻喉]听力测定；[耳鼻喉]听力测验法
deletion	[dɪˈliːʃən]	*n.* 删除；[遗]缺失；删除部分
ptosis	[ˈtəʊsɪs] (*pl.* ptoses)	*n.* [医]下垂；上睑下垂；下垂症
dysarthria	[dɪsˈɑːθrɪə]	*n.* [耳鼻喉]构音障碍；构音困难
cerebellar ataxia		小脑性共济失调；小脑运动失调
external ophthalmoplegia		眼外肌麻痹，外眼肌瘫痪；眼外肌瘫痪，外眼肌麻痹

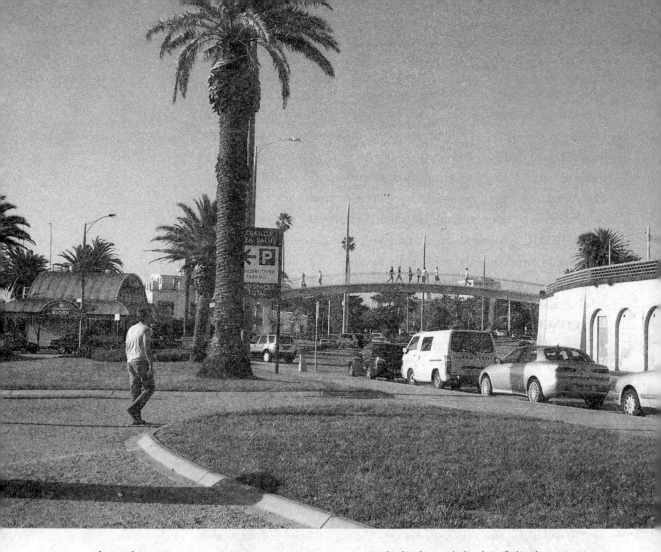

buccal mucosa   颊黏膜，口腔黏膜，唇粘膜

◆ Questions

1. Why should all patients with the combination of deafness and diabetes presenting to diabetes clinics be screened for the m. 3243A>G mutation?

2. Can we decide that those patients present no mitochondrial disease，if the screening test for the m. 3243A>G mutation is negative?

3. What other clinical features of mitochondrial disease could be presented besides deafness?

4. Why did the author think that we underestimate the prevalence of diabetes and deafness due to mtDNA mutations?

5. How can we ensure that patients harboring mtDNA mutations are correctly diagnosed?

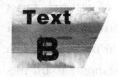

Prevalence of Gestational Diabetes Mellitus (GDM) and Its Outcomes in Jammu Region

Preeti Wahi

Abstract

Introduction: The present study seeks to evaluate the prevalence and outcomes of gestational diabetes mellitus (GDM) from Jammu region.

Methods: During the period of study, women at 24th to 28th week of gestation were investigated for the presence of (GDM) according to Diabetes In Pregnancy Study Group India (guidelines). The maternal and fetal outcomes were recorded and compared with (a) non-diabetic control group and (b) non-interventional untreated GDM group.

Results: The overall prevalence of GDM was found to be 6.94%. In the untreated group, family history of diabetes was 24.19%, caesarean section 22.58% and preterm delivery 16.13%, whereas the prevalence of macrosomia was 16.2% and shoulder dystocia 6.45%. These figures were found to be significantly higher when compared to the data obtained from the treated GDM group which was as follows: caesarean section 8.5%, preterm delivery 4.2%, macrosomia 10% and shoulder dystocia 1.2%.

Conclusion: The study emphasizes the importance of screening for GDM and timely optimum intervention for a significant positive effect on both maternal as well as foetal outcomes in pregnancy. This also builds a strong case for adherence to DIPSI guidelines in diagnosis and management of GDM.

Introduction

Very little data is available from the Jammu region with regard to the prevalence of gestational diabetes mellitus (GDM). This is quite unbecoming considering the fact that a lot of research focus today is on the well-being of mother and the newborn child in general and in the situation of GDM or diabetes mellitus in particular. The present study, therefore, attempts to elicit valuable inputs to fill this void and was based in Government Medical College Hospital, which is one of the largest public sector hospitals in north India catering to patients from different parts of the Jammu region.

In the Indian context, screening is essential in all pregnant women as the Indian women have eleven-fold increased risk of developing glucose intolerance during pregnancy compared to Caucasian women. The present study, therefore, has compiled authentic data regarding the prevalence of GDM from Jammu region and its effect on pregnancy outcomes.

The information, inferences and conclusions drawn from this study are expected to be pooled with similar information from other parts of country and thus prove vital in formulating effective and timely allocation of resources to improve pregnancy outcomes in diabetics and at the same time prevent morbidity and mortality in diabetic pregnant women and their offspring.

The present study followed the DIPSI (Diabetesin Pregnancy Study Group India) guidelines for screening of our subjects so that a uniform common protocol followed by similar study groups in other parts of the country could enable a fair and judicious correlation with each other. Besides, DIPSI guidelines also facilitate both economical and feasible mode of evaluation. One of the important guidelines of DIPSI was to put the GDM patient on treatment (MNT/MNT + Insulin Therapy). Unfortunately, some of the patients refused to follow this guideline because of the strong traditional belief that restriction of diet will affect the robust development of the fetus. We utilized this "default" group of patients for comparison with the patients who were put on treatment so as to see the effect of these two groups i. e. who received treatment with those who did not receive any treatment.

Material and Methods

The present prospective study was conducted on patients in chronological order attending the antenatal clinics in the Department of Gynaecology and Obstetrics, SMGS Hospital in association with the Department of General Medicine, Government Medical College and Hospital, Jammu for a period of one year with effect from

December, 2007 to November, 2008. During the period of study, subjects at 24th to 28th week of gestation were evaluated for presence of GDM according to DIPSI recommended method and followed-up to determine the outcomes of pregnancy as perpredesigned proforma.

The inclusion criteria included pregnant women at 24th to 28th week of gestation, while cases pertaining to type 1 diabetes mellitus, urinary tract infection (UTI), major chronic diseases like carcinoma, tuberculosis and diseases leading to accumulation of fluid and appearance of protein in urine like congestive cardiac failure (CCF), renal failure and advanced liver failure were excluded from the present study.

Diagnosis of GDM: This criterion was established if 2-hour venous plasma glucose after 75-g of oral glucose load in fasting state $\geqslant$140 mg/dl.

Results

A total of 2025 subjects at 24th to 28th weeks of gestation, attending the antenatal clinics of Department of Gynaecology and Obstetrics, SMGS Hospital, Government Medical College, Jammu, were evaluated for GDM according to DIPSI recommended method. Out of 2025 subjects, 132 (6.51%) were diagnosed as GDM. This study group was divided into two parts: Group Ⅰ were those who did not receive any treatment (n=62). Group Ⅱ were those who received treatment in form of MNT/MNT+Insulin Therapy (n=70). One hundred and forty (140) non-diabetic pregnant ladies were included as control in our study. Among the 70 GDM subjects who received treatment, 44 (61.91%) were put on MNT and 26 (38.09%) were put on MNT+Insulin Therapy.

Discussion

The present prospective hospital-based study, which was the first of its kind to be undertaken in this part of the country, showed the prevalence of GDM as 6.94%. GDM prevalence has been reported variably from 1.4% to 14% worldwide and differently among racial and ethnic groups. Prevalence is higher in Blacks, Latinos, Native Americans and Asian women than White women. A similar study in Kashmiri women from same state gave a prevalence figure of 3.8%.

Diabetes mellitus is an epidemically explosive problem which is increasing at an unstoppable pace. DIPSI guideline having suggested one time plasma sugar level as a measure to detect GDM is an attempt to preempt future possibility and predisposition for diabetes mellitus.

Our findings of this study are largely at tandem with those of literature at the national as well as international level. We, therefore, infer from the above study that Jammu region is, despite its varying ethnicity, food habits, terrain and living standard, very much a part of diabetes spectrum the world over.

Secondly, treatment right after detection of GDM state is effective in stemming the adverse pregnancy outcomes largely in terms of preterm, macrosomia, gestational hypertension and shoulder dystocia which are statistically significant.

Still birth and rDS complications in pregnancy were not affected significantly which may be because of this being a hospital-based study where proper follow-up and patient care are excellent.

Compared with women of normal OGTT, women with GDM were older. Mean age$\pm$SD in GDM group was 27.2$\pm$2.3 years, while in control group it was 26.2$\pm$2.3 years. Similar study from South India showed age$>$25 years as a risk factor for GDM. This finding is in agreement with the result of other studies conducted in Indian subcontinent.

In our study, a significant proportion of subjects with GDM were overweight [19 (30.65%)] and obese [16 (25.8%)]. Study of prevalence of GDM in Southern Iran (Bander Aban City) showed that BMI of 25 kg/m^2 or more were significantly more prevalent in GDM subjects 7 which is in accordance with the present study. GDM was seen to be least prevalent (3.23%) in underweight subjects (BMI$<$18.5 kg/m^2).

We observed family history of diabetes mellitus in significant proportion of cases i. e. 15 (24.19%). A study from Tamil Nadu also concluded that family history of diabetes was significant risk factor for GDM. This finding is in accordance with studies in Europe that showed positive family history of type-2 diabetes in majority of subjects with GDM.

Our study revealed that the most common complications seen in GDM mothers was gestational hypertension (6.45%), followed by postpartum haemorrhage (3%), abortion (2.7%) and premature rupture of membranes (1.6%). The prospective cohort study performed in 1,310 women in Iran showed the most common maternal complication was gestational hypertension (9.7%). Another study of 972 GDM mothers in Saudi Arabia showed that common complications were perineal tear (18%) that causes postpartum haemorrhage, followed by gestational hypertension (2%).

In the present study, 22.58% of non-intervention GDM ladies delivered via caesarean section while only 8.5% of treatment GDM ladies delivered via caesarean section and the difference between the two groups is statistically significant (p = 0.04). A research-controlled trial was done which studied the effect of treatment on GDM pregnant ladies and found that induction of labour was less in treated group than in non-treated group (p<0.001), however rate of caesarean section was same. Also, when non-intervention group was compared to control, again the difference is statistically significant (p=0.04).

A Chennai based study of GDM ladies also shows that assisted deliveries were significantly higher among GDM group than controls (p<0.001).

Our study demonstrated that 14.52% of newborns of GDM mothers in non-treatment group were macrosomics while the figure was 10% in treated group (p=0.02, c^2=5.19) and 7% in control population (p=0.01, c^2=4.53).

Most of the studies shows fetal macrosomia in 10%—20% of infants born to GDM mothers. 11 Asian Indian mothers also show prevalence of large babies as 27.6% in GDM group.

In Australia based study, obstetric outcomes of 138 treated GDM ladies were studied and found that treated GDM had 8% macrosomic rate which was significantly less (p=0.02) than rate of 17% in control population.

Similar results were obtained in USA based study where incidence of macrosomia was reduced in intervention group as compared to routine care group (10% vs 20%, p=0.001).

Our study showed that prevalence of still birth and respiratory distress syndrome is 4.84% and 3.23% in untreated group while none in treated and control population. The difference between the two groups is not statistically significant. A similar study from Thailand showed incidence of respiratory distress syndrome as 4.9% and 1.2%, respectively.

Also, the prevalence of shoulder dystocia in untreated diabetic population was 9.6% which is significantly higher than in treated group (1.4%, p=0.03) and control group (4%, p=0.03). This is supported by a British-based study on GDM population where it was stated that in females who were treated for GDM, shoulder dystocia was significantly less common (odd's ratio 0.40, 95% confidence interval 0.21—0.75).

GDM is like a natural IGTT. DIPSI guidelines come out with a major breakthrough by detecting such state with single prick thereby facilitating a very quick and non-tedious method to pick out such conditions.

As many follow-up studies come in from various states in India and other third-world countries, this methodology can be integrated into national program to detect GDM and stop its unfettered growth.

Conclusion

The study evidently proves the advantage of adhering to DIPSI guidelines in diagnosis and management of GDM for a significantly positive effect on pregnancy outcomes both in relation to mother as well the child.

Acknowledgement

The authors are highly thankful to the Postgraduate Departments of Medicine, Obstetrics and Gynaecology and PSM Government Medical College, Jammu for providing adequate facilities for working on this study.

(2210 words)

※ The text is extracted from *JAPI*, April, 2011, Vol. 59.

References

1. Dornhost A, Paterson C M, Nicholls J S et al. High prevalence of GDM in women from ethnic minority groups. Diabetic Med 1992, 9:820 – 822.
2. Zargar A H, Sheikh M I, Bashir M I, Masoodi S R, Laway B A, Warsi A I, Bhat M H, Dar F A. Prevalence of gestational diabetes mellitusin Kashmiri women from the Indian subcontinent. Diabetes Res ClinPract 2004, 66:139 – 145.
3. Seshiah V, Balaji V, Balaji M S et al. Prevalence of gestational diabetes mellitus in South India (Tamil Nadu)—a community-based study. J Assoc Physicians India 2008, 56:329 – 333.
4. Sribaddana S H, Deshaband R, Rajapalase D, Silva K, Fernando D J. The prevalence of gestational diabetes in a Sri Lankan antenatal clinic. Ceylon Med J

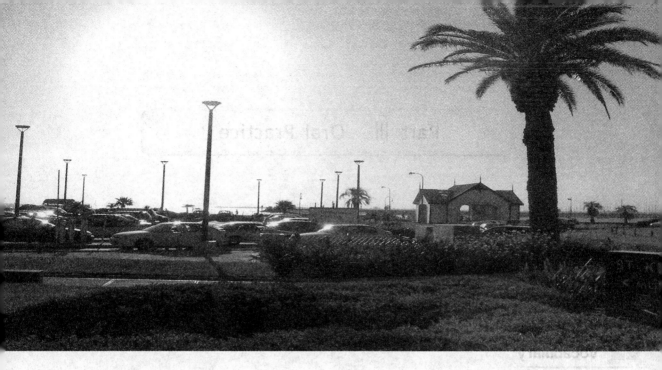

1998, 43:88 - 91.

5. Seshiah V, Balaji V, Balaji M S, Sanjeevi C B, Green A. Gestational diabetes mellitus in India. J Assoc Physicians India 2004, 52:707 - 711.

6. Hadaegh F, Tohidi M, Harati H, Kharandish M, Rahimi S. Prevalence of gestational diabetes mellitus in Southern Iran (BandarAbbas City). Endocr Pract 2005, 11:313 - 318.

7. Kautzky-Willer A, Bancher-Todesca D. Gestational diabetes. Wien Med Wochenschr 2003, 153:478 - 484.

8. Keshavarz M, Cheung N W, Babaee G R et al. Gestational diabetes in Iran: incidence, risk factors and pregnancy outcomes. Diabetes Res Clin Pract 2005, 69: 279 - 286.

9. Mallah K, Narchi H, Kulaylat N A, Shaban M S. Gestational and pre-gestational diabetes: comparison of maternal and fetal characteristics and outcome. Int J Gynecol Obstet 1997, 58:203 - 209.

10. Pennison E, Egerman R S. Perinatal outcomes in gestational diabetes: a comparison of criteria for diagnosis. Am J Obstet Gynecol 2001, 184:1118 - 1121.

11. Shefali A K, Kavitha M, Deepa R, Mohan V. Pregnancy outcomes in pre-gestational and gestational diabetic women in comparison tonon-diabetic women—a prospective study in Asian Indian mothers (CUrES - 35). J Assoc Physicians India 2006, 54:613 - 618.

12. Moses R G, Griffiths R D. Can a diagnosis of gestational diabetes bean advantage to the outcome of pregnancy? Journal of the Society for Gynecology Investigation, 1995, 2:523 - 525. From http://care. diabetesjournals. org.

Practice 1
Clinical Inquiry—Department of Respiratory System

 Vocabulary

laryngeal	[ləˈrɪndʒɪəl]	*adj.* 喉的；喉头治疗用的 of or relating to the larynx
obstruction	[əbˈstrʌkʃ(ə)n]	*n.* 阻塞，梗阻
emergent	[ɪˈmɜːdʒənt]	*adj.* 紧急的
lesion	[ˈliːʒ(ə)n]	*n.* （因伤病而致的）损伤，损害；病变 damage to someone's skin or part of their body such as their stomach or brain, caused by injury or illness
inhale	[ɪnˈheɪl]	*v.* 吸入；吸气 When you inhale, you breathe in. When you inhale something such as smoke, you take it into your lungs when you breathe in
aggravation	[ˌægrəˈveʃən]	*n.* 加剧，加重
sputum	[ˈspjʊtəm]	*n.* [生理]痰；唾液 liquid in your mouth which you have coughed up from your lungs
tracheotomy	[ˌtreɪkɪˈɒtəmɪ]	*n.* 气管切开术 an operation to cut a hole in someone's throat so that they can breathe
dyspnea	[dɪspˈnɪə]	*n.* [内科]呼吸困难 difficulty in breathing or in catching the breath
stridor	[ˈstraɪdə]	*n.* 喘鸣 a high-pitched whistling sound made during respiration, caused by obstruction of the air passages
thorax	[ˈθɒræks]	*n.* 胸（部）；胸廓 the part of your body between your neck and diaphragm (area just above your stomach)
hypoxia	[haɪˈpɒksɪə]	*n.* （组织）缺氧 deficiency in the amount of oxygen delivered to the body tissues
complexion	[kəmˈplekʃən]	*n.* 面色，面容，气色 the natural color or appearance of the skin on your face
cyanosis	[ˌsaɪəˈnəʊsɪs]	*n.* 发绀，青紫 a bluish-purple discoloration of skin

		and mucous membranes usually resulting from a deficiency of oxygen in the blood
arrhythmia	[əˈrɪðmɪə]	*n.* [内科]心律失常,心律不整 any variation from the normal rhythm in the heartbeat
incontinence	[ɪnˈkɒntɪnəns]	*n.* (大小便)失禁 inability to control urine or feces from coming out of your body
suffocation	[ˌsʌfəˈkeɪʃn]	*n.* 窒息;闷死
recumbent	[rɪˈkʌmbənt]	*adj.* 躺着的,仰卧的;侧卧的 lying down on your back or side
anesthesia	[ˌænəsˈθɪʒə]	*n.* 麻醉;麻木

 ## Using Lay Terms in Explanations

Explanations should be given in words the patients will understand, avoiding medical terms. Using lay terms—words familiar to people without medical knowledge—can help patients understand explanations. e. g. :

Medical Terms	Lay Terms
1. larynx	throat
2. lesion	damage
3. inhale	suck/breathe in
4. aggravate	worsen
5. sputum	phlegm
6. dyspnea	difficulty in breathing
7. suffocate	choke
8. anesthesia	numbness

Sample Dialogue

(A nursing round for a patient with laryngeal obstruction)

Nurse A: Laryngeal obstruction is one of the emergent diseases due to the throat or its vicinal tissue lesion in the ENT department. It can cause breathing difficulty. How to receive the patient with laryngeal obstruction and match the aid are very important. So today we are talking about the nursing of laryngeal obstruction. I hope our new colleagues will get good command of receiving patients with laryngeal obstruction.

Nurse A: Firstly, let us ask nurse B to give an introduction of the medical history.

Nurse B: Wang Hua, male, 55 years old. Six months ago, he had a hoarse voice and a sensation of swallowing with foreign bodies, without apparent causes. These symptoms became more serious gradually. Three days ago, he was admitted because of inhaling breathing difficulty with progressive aggravation as an emergency case. Admission diagnosis: tumor of larynx and breathing difficulty in degree two.

Nurse A: What preparations we should do when we get a call to receive a patient with laryngeal obstruction?

Nurse C: We should prepare a bed, oxygen delivery, aspiration of sputum, tracheotomy package and tracheal casing pipes.

Nurse A: The key point is how to evaluate the degree of the difficulty in breathing. How can we define the degree of the difficulty in breathing? What's the difference when we treat patients with the difficulty in breathing in different degrees?

Nurse D: According to the patient's condition, it can be divided into four degrees. The first degree: the patient shows no dyspnea when he is quiet and mild inspiratory dyspnea and laryngeal stridor when he is activating or crying. The second degree: the patient shows mild inspiratory dyspnea and laryngeal stridor with dented soft tissue around thorax when inspirating. These will aggravate when he is activating but with no effect on sleep and diets. The third degree: the patient shows obvious difficulty in breathing and louder laryngeal stridor with significant dented soft tissue around thorax when inspiriting. He also appears to have some hypoxia symptoms: being restless, uneasy to fall asleep, less appetite for food and speeded-up pulse. The fourth degree: the patient has extreme difficulty in breathing. He is extremely restless with a pale complexion or cyanosis, he shows arrhythmias, coma, incontinence, etc., which will result in death due to suffocation without timely rescue.

Nurse A: This patient shows dyspnea with second degree, and our principles of treatments are to strengthen intensive observation of the disease and to prepare for the tracheotomy. Then, what specific nursing treatment should be taken?

Nurse F: We can take the following procedures: 1. Keep the patient in semi recumbent position or sitting position. 2. Let the patient have oxygen uptake. 3. Relax the patient to avoid the dyspnea caused by excessive tension. 4. Keep intensive observation of the patient's vital signs, the color of his lip and nail bed, three dented states and change of blood oxygen concentration. 5. Prepare and cooperate with doctor to take the tracheotomy: (a) Blood drawing for emergency check. (b) Establish the vein passage. (c) If the tracheotomy was taken under local anesthesia by the bed, we must help to pose the patient (lying position without pillow), prepare lights, objects and effective vacuum suction in the operation. (d) If the tracheotomy was taken under general anesthesia in OR, we must tell the patient not to drink and eat.

Nurse A: Today, we are talking about the procedures to receive the patient with laryngeal obstruction and the matching aid. Through this round, I hope that everyone can understand the clinical classification of the degrees of breathing difficulty and its treatment principles. We should focus on the receiving and nursing of patients with laryngeal obstruction to boost our quality of care and the effect of rescue. Thank you for participating in the nursing rounds!

Activities and Role-play (inviting students to improvise and act it out)

Practice 2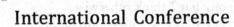

International Conference
—Discussion and Showing Comments

 Useful Expressions for Discussion

1. I'd like to preface my remarks with a description of … (with some general statements about …)
2. The first point I'd like to make about … is …
3. We'll shift to the topic of …
4. That brings me to the second point.
5. Let's go back again to what each of us considers important.
6. Now let's move on to the next point.
7. I'd like to go to some details about this point.
8. Since this point is very important to us, I'd like to spend some time describing it in greater details.
9. I'd like to discuss this in depth.
10. I don't feel that I should go into experimental details, since they are published.

 Useful Expressions for Showing Approval

1. That would be absolutely true.
2. I can't agree more.

3. That is exactly what I mean.

4. I think that could be the correct assumption.

5. I do not deny the possibility of A's being involved in B.

6. I'm in complete agreement with you on that point.

7. I'm completely in concurrence with Mr. A in this point.

8. I share Mr. A's comments about this point.

9. I have no objection to extending our theory.

10. I'm not in disagreement with you on this point.

 ## Useful Expressions for Showing Disapproval

1. I hope not.

2. I don't think so.

3. I'm sorry I must disagree with Mr. A on that point.

4. I am not sure I can agree with your statement about that.

5. I respect your opinion, but I think otherwise.

6. You may be right, but I view it a little differently.

7. The difference between our opinions is too wide to be easily changed.

8. I doubt that the test samples become available so soon.

9. I differ with you on this point.

10. I would be strongly opposed to that proposal.

 ## Useful Expressions for Showing Comments

1. I'd like to make a few comments to clarify some of those points made earlier that I believe might be misunderstood.

2. If I might be permitted to make a comment, I would like to say that this sample may not be suitable for the studies.

3. Another comment I'd like to make is that this substance is sparingly soluble in water.

4. To comment on Dr. A's question, we have observed a similar effect of A on B.

5. I just want to remark on the last point Mr. A made.

6. I'd like to present my opinion on this point.

7. I'd like to place emphasis on the face that no drug is absolutely safe.

8. This is an extremely important point that nobody should forget.

9. We have enough reason to believe that those men would be sensitive to the stimuli.

10. I feel strongly that the results should be viewed as a great advance in this field.

Activities and Role-play (inviting students to improvise and act it out)

Practice 3 ||||

Oral English for Culture and on Social Occasions
—Chinese Scenic Spots and Historical Sites

 Occasion: Tourism Agency

Useful Expressions for Tourism Inquiry

1. Excuse me. Could you tell me where the tourist information center is?
2. Can you recommend a hotel which is not too expensive?
3. I'd like to stay at a hotel near the beach. Would you recommend one?
4. Please tell me about some interesting places in this city.
5. Excuse me. May I have a free city map?
6. Please give me a sightseer's pamphlet.
7. How much is the Shangri-La tour for 7 days?
8. We particularly want to visit Beijing, Xi'an and Shanghai. Do you have any tour including all these places?
9. Here are the brochures that describe various tour routes in China. You can choose anyone you like.
10. What famous scenic spots does this city have?

Activities and Role-play (inviting students to improvise and act it out)

Useful Expressions for Visiting Scenic Spots and Historical Sites

1. A week may be spent in seeing the interesting sights of the city.
2. They spent the whole day wandering about seeing the sights.
3. I'm afraid two days isn't enough for you to see all the places of interest.
4. The tourist area is dotted with historic and scenic attractions.

5. The island abounds with places of historic and scenic interest.

6. Yueyang Tower Pavilion is a famous scenic spot in the Dongting Lake area.

7. The Summer Palace is the largest and the best preserved of the imperial gardens in China.

8. I suppose we'd better go to famous Yuyuan Garden which is located in the southern part of the city of Shanghai.

9. Visitors are struck by its ingenious architecture and exotic layout.

10. The dragon's head is beautifully modeled and is rising proudly over there.

Names for Some Chinese Scenic Spots and Historical Sites

北海公园	Beihai Park
故宫博物院	the Palace Museum
革命历史博物馆	the Museum of Revolutionary History
天安门广场	Tian'anmen Square
毛主席纪念堂	Chairman Mao Zedong Memorial Hall
保和殿	the Hall of Preserving Harmony
中和殿	the Hall of Central Harmony
长城	the Great Wall
午门	the Meridian Gate
紫金山天文台	Purple Mountain Observatory
紫禁城	the Forbidden City
御花园	Imperial Garden
颐和园	Summer Palace
天坛	Temple of Heaven
周口店遗址	Zhoukoudian Ancient Site
太和殿	the Hall of Supreme Harmony
祈年殿	the Hall of Prayer for Good Harvest
烽火台	the Beacon Tower
人民大会堂	the Great Hall of the People
清东陵	Eastern Royal Tombs of the Qing Dynasty
乾清宫	Palace of Heavenly Purity
民族文化宫	the Cultural Palace for Nationalities
劳动人民文化宫	Working People's Cultural Palace
北京工人体育馆	Beijing Worker's Stadium
仙人洞	Fairy Cave
黄果树瀑布	Huangguoshu Falls
苏州园林	Suzhou Gardens
西山晴雪	the Sunny Western Hills after Snow

避暑山庄	the Imperial Mountain Summer Resort
龙门石窟	Longmen Stone Cave
庐山	Lushan Mountain
天池	Heaven Pool
蓬莱水城	Penglai Water City
大雁塔	Big Wild Goose Pagoda
华山	Huashan Mountain
峨嵋山	Emei Mountain
石林	Stone Forest
白马寺	White Horse Temple
白云山	White Cloud Mountain
布达拉宫	Potala Palace
大运河	Grand Canal
滇池	Dianchi Lake
杜甫草堂	Du Fu Cottage
都江堰	Dujiang Dam
鼓浪屿	Gulangyu Islet
观音阁	Goddess of Mercy Pavilion
归元寺	Guiyuan Buddhist Temple
甘露寺	Sweet Dew Temple
黄花岗七十二烈士墓	Mausoleum of the 72 Martyrs
华清池	Huaqing Hot Spring
昭君墓	Zhaojun's Tomb
毛泽东故居	Mao Zedong's former Residence
周恩来故居	Zhou Enlai's former Residence
越秀公园	Yuexiu Park
岳阳楼	Yueyang Tower
南湖公园	South Lake Park
中山公园	Zhongshan Park
武侯祠	Temple of Marquis Wu
漓江	Lijiang River
寒山寺	Hanshan Temple
静心斋	Heart-East Study
黄鹤楼	Yellow Crane Tower
黄山	Huangshan Mountain
天下第一关	the First Pass Under Heaven
桂林山水	Guilin Scenery with Hills and Waters
秦始皇兵马俑	The Terracotta Army

References for Further Discussion

1. The Forbidden City

The Forbidden City was the Chinese imperial palace from the mid-Ming Dynasty to the end of the Qing Dynasty. It is located in the middle of Beijing, China and now houses the Palace Museum. For almost five centuries, it served as the home of the Emperor and his household, and the ceremonial and political center of Chinese government.

2. The Great Wall

The Great Wall of China is a series of stone and earthen fortifications in China, built, rebuilt, and maintained between the 6th century BC and the 16th century to protect the northern borders of the Chinese Empire during the rule of successive dynasties. Several walls, referred to as the Great Wall of China, were built since the 5th century BC. The most famous is the wall built between 220 BC—200 BC by the first Emperor of China, Qin Shi Huang; little of it remains; it was much farther north than the current wall, which was built during the Ming Dynasty.

3. The Terracotta Army

The Terracotta Army is the Terracotta Warriors and Horses of Shi Huang Di, the First Emperor of China. The terracotta figures, dating from 210 BC, were discovered in 1974 by several local farmers near Xi'an, Shaanxi province, China, near the Mausoleum of the First Qin Emperor. The figures vary in height (184—197 cm), according to their role, the tallest being the Generals. The figures include warriors, chariots, horses, officials, acrobats, strongmen, and musicians. Current estimates are that in the three pits containing the Terracotta Army there were over 8,000 soldiers, 130 chariots with 520 horses and 150 cavalry horses, the majority still buried in the pits.

4. Mount Tai

Mount Tai is a mountain of historical and cultural significance located north of the city of Tai'an, in Shandong Province, China. The tallest peak is Jade Emperor Peak, which is commonly reported as 1545 meters (5069 feet) tall, but is described by the Chinese government as 1532. 7 meters (5028. 5 feet). Mount Tai is one of the "Five Sacred Mountains of Taoism". It is associated with sunrise, birth, and renewal, and is often regarded the foremost of the five. The temples on its slopes have been a destination for pilgrims for 3,000 years.

5. The Huangshan Mountain

The Huangshan Mountain (Yellow Mountain) is a mountain range in southern Anhui province in eastern China. The area is very famous for its scenic beauty, which lies in the peculiar shapes of the granite peaks, in the weather-shaped Huangshan Pine trees, and in views of the clouds from above. The area also has hot springs and natural pools. Today, it is a UNESCO World Heritage Site and one of China's most popular tourist destinations.

Unit 4

Key Points

Learning Targets

- To master the skill of *taking notes while listening*
- To learn the skill of *analyzing the global structure of a passage*
- To learn about the academic terms of gastric carcinoma in clinical diagnostic conversation

Learning Focus

- How to do opening remarks and introduce lecturers at an international academic conference

Cultural Points

- Concepts of a modern city

✓音、视频资源
✓参考译文
✓参考答案
✓学术探讨

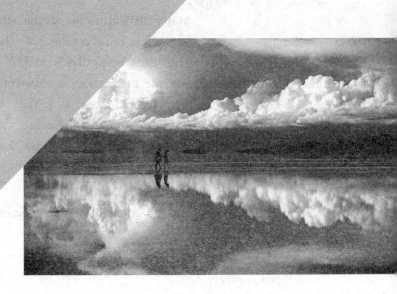

Part Ⅰ   Listening Comprehension

Video 1

The Presentation on Influenza Vaccines

Exercise Ⅰ   The list below includes types of analyses used for vaccine strain selection. Which two are not mentioned by the speaker?

    A. Virus neutralization tests

    B. Hemagglutination inhibition tests

    C. Epidemiological analysis

    D. Antigenic cartography

    E. Candidate strain effectiveness

    F. HA and NA gene phylogenetic analyses

    1. _____ _____

Exercise Ⅱ   Complete the summary below. Choose no more than two words from the speech for each answer.

Major difficulties for vaccine strain selection

    Firstly, vaccine effectiveness relies on the __2__ between HA of the vaccines and HA of virus circulating strains. But the antibody to HA in linked to __3__. Secondly, the timetable for influenza vaccine production is comparatively __4__. Usually the vaccines have to be available in February or March, i. e. the __5__ in northern hemisphere. Then, the __6__ which is known as candidate vaccine virus should be proper for vaccine production and easy for the manufacturers to grow. Lastly, it is also important to choose the strain specific reagents required in __7__.

Exercise Ⅲ   Decide whether the following statements are true (T), false (F) or not given (NG).

    8. The different steps in manufacturing seasonal influenza vaccines are all linked with one another.

    9. The antigenic analysis is operated in different ways from that for isolated vaccine

virus strains.

10. There are much more licensed quadrivalent influenza vaccines than the past in America.

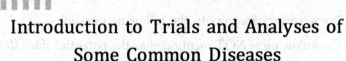

Introduction to Trials and Analyses of Some Common Diseases

Exercise I Take notes while watching the video, and then complete the following sentences.

In this figure, we have all the different conditions along the X-axis and DALYs per trial and you can see overall there's __1__ in the study of diseases. There is a range of __2__ to __3__ DALYs per trial, which represents a greater than __4__ per range in DALYs per trial. So what this indicates is that in allocating our resources and our research activity, certainly the burden of disease is not the __5__ factor. There are other determinants of what we choose to study.

Not surprisingly, the correlation was __6__, so the Spearman's correlation factor was 0.5 between research activity and disease burden. So this was DALYs per trial.

Exercise II Decide whether the following statements are true (T) or false (F).

7. Compared with leukemia, lung cancer is underrepresented due to its higher number of DALYs.

8. The more number of trials, the higher number of DALYs.

9. The number of trials, degree of disease burden and DALYs per trial are correlated with one other.

10. The purpose of introducing DALYs per trial is to assess the conformity between research activity and actual disease burden.

11. Disease burden explains why there is difference in the number of participants and sample size in a clinical trial.

12. Ischemic heart disease and stroke are two most underrepresented diseases with the heaviest disease burden in elderly patients.

Listening 1
Study: Stop-Smoking Aid Ups Cardiovascular Risks

Exercise Ⅰ   Choose correct answers to the following questions.

1. Which of the following is NOT mentioned as the potential side effects of taking the drug Chantix?
   - A. heart failure
   - B. heart rhythm irregularities
   - C. stroke
   - D. gastritis

2. Which of the following statements is NOT true?
   - A. Professor Sonal Singh was a leading author of the study.
   - B. In total, 8200 smokers from around the world participated in the studies when the studies began.
   - C. The risk of heart problems among study participants who took the smoking cessation drug was lower than that of cardiovascular disease in the placebo groups.
   - D. The heart problems began to show up as early as one year after the volunteers completed a 12-week course of treatment with Chantix.

3. What will the company (Chantix's producer) do in the future?
   - A. refuse to work with the FDA to do safety analysis
   - B. possibly add a warning about cardiovascular problems to the black box
   - C. accuse the researchers of their studies
   - D. fail to pass the pre-approval of Chantix

Exercise Ⅱ   Listen and try to fill in the blanks with the exact words you hear.

Ⅰ. The study reviewed the data from 14 of __4__ Chantix. It found a 72-percent increase in the risk of cardiovascular __5__ among smokers who took the quit-smoking aid compared to those who received a placebo or sugar pill. Researchers evaluated information collected on 8,200 smokers from around the world who did not have __6__ when the studies began.

Ⅱ. While the __7__ may not sound significant, Singh says the impact is great if you consider the number of users in the US and nearly 100 countries worldwide where Chantix has been approved as a __8__.

Ⅲ. So, even a small __9__ increase in relative risk of heart attack translates into thousands of __10__ in the United States. And if you look at 13 million users of

Chantix worldwide even that ___11___ of a percent risk—you're talking about thousands of lives.

Listening 2 ||||

Study Links Everyday Chemicals to Obesity

Exercise I   Listen and try to fill in the blanks with the exact words you hear.

I. About half of the world's population is overweight or ___1___. And, scientists and policy makers say the problem is growing and causing people to die ___2___ because of obesity-related illnesses such as ___3___ and heart disease.

II. The scientists agree eating too much and exercising too little remain the ___4___ of obesity. But they cite new evidence that mice exposed to ___5___ disrupting chemicals during ___6___ produce offspring that became fat as adults.

III. The scientists agree obesity is caused by ___7___ factors and must be treated in multiple ways. They say new research shows obese patients can achieve ___8___ weight loss without drugs using a low-cost approach involving innovative intensive ___9___.

Exercise II   Decide whether the following statements are true (T) or false (F).

10. Studies found that exposure to certain substances during development, neither in the womb nor during infancy, may lead to obesity later in life.

11. Scientists agree that eating too much and exercising too little are still the two significant causes of obesity.

12. Tributylin may presumably get people fatter through altering metabolism.

13. Beverly Rubin says people can do little to avoid exposure to hormone-altering chemicals.

14. If pregnant mothers are exposed to sources that contain this Bisphenol A leaching, it results in worst impact during development, during early development, during fetal development.

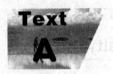

Text
A

Address at the WHO Congress on Traditional Medicine

Dr Margaret Chan
(Director-General of the World Health Organization)

Dr Chen, honorable ministers, distinguished guests, ladies and gentlemen,

First and foremost, let me say how pleased I am to be in Beijing to address this WHO congress on traditional medicine. I also want to extend my thanks to the Chinese Ministry of Health and the State Administration of Traditional Chinese Medicine for co-hosting the event together with WHO.

I will speak about traditional medicine in three contexts: the current reality, the renewal of primary health care, and the rise of chronic diseases. In doing so, I will focus on how each of these contexts provides some compelling reasons to make better use of traditional medicine and its practitioners.

I will also speak about some of the challenges faced in efforts to bring traditional medicine into the mainstream of health care, appropriately, effectively, and above all safely.

Let me begin with the current reality, which on at least one level, is quite straightforward. Traditional medicine is generally available, affordable, and commonly used in large parts of Africa, Asia, and Latin America.

For many millions of people, often living in rural areas of developing countries, herbal medicines, traditional treatments, and traditional practitioners are the main—sometimes the only source of health care.

This is care that is close to homes, accessible, and affordable. In some systems of traditional medicine, such as traditional Chinese medicine and the Ayurveda system historically rooted in India, traditional practices are supported by wisdom and experience acquired over centuries.

In these contexts where traditional medicine has strong historical and cultural roots, practitioners are usually well-known members of the community who command respect and are supported by public confidence in their abilities and remedies.

This is the reality, and this form of care unquestionably soothes, treats many ailments, reduces suffering, and relieves pain. This is the reality, but it is not the ideal.

When we see estimates that around 60% of young children in some African countries suffering from high fever, presumably caused by malaria, are treated at home with herbal remedies, we have a very serious problem. Malaria can kill within 24 hours. Modern drugs can greatly improve the prospects of survival.

During this year, WHO estimates that around 136 million women will give birth. Of these women, around 58 million will receive no medical assistance whatsoever during childbirth and the postpartum period, endangering their lives and that of their infants.

Again, we have a very serious problem. The consensus is now solid. The stubbornly high numbers of maternal deaths will not go down until more women have killed attendants at birth and access to emergency obstetric care.

The point I wish to make is straightforward. Traditional medicine has much to offer, but it cannot always substitute for access to highly effective modern drugs and emergency measures that make such a critical life-and-death difference for many millions of people.

This is not a criticism of traditional medicine. This is a failure of health systems in many countries to deliver effective interventions to those in greatest need, on an adequate scale. In the context of the drive to meet the health-related Millennium Development Goals, this failure is now widely acknowledged. Intensive efforts are under way to correct this failure, to strengthen basic health infrastructures, services, and staff.

But there is another side to the current reality, and this is also indicative of inadequacies in the way our world is delivering health care. This is the striking increase, in affluent societies, in the popularity of treatments and remedies that complement orthodox medicine or sometimes serve as an alternative to conventional treatments.

Recent studies conducted in North America and Europe indicate that these remedies tend to be used most in groups with higher incomes and higher levels of education. In many cases, the costs are not covered by medical insurance schemes. The use of these complementary and alternative therapies has become a multi-billion dollar industry that is expected to continue its rapid growth. This is not the poor man's alternative to conventional care.

What does this trend represent? The reaction of the medical establishment is predictable and, I believe, largely legitimate. This trend has some dangers.

As I said, some systems of traditional medicine have histories dating back thousands of years. Over a comparatively short period of time, modern medicine has developed powerful methodologies for proving efficacy, ensuring quality, standardizing good manufacturing practices, testing for safety, and conducting post-marketing surveillance for adverse effects.

Many, but not all, traditional medicines have an inadequate evidence base when measured by these standards. Tests for quality and standards for production tend to be less rigorous and controlled. Products may escape the strict regulations set up to ensure drug safety. Practitioners may not be certified or licensed.

These concerns are legitimate, but we are still left with a central question: what explains the sharp rise in the use of complementary and alternative medicines? Again, we can turn to the medical establishment for some explanations. Some commentators in journals such as the *British Medical Journal*, *The Lancet*, and the *New England Journal of Medicine* interpret this trend as a biting criticism of high-technology, specialized medicine, despite all its well-documented merits.

Medical care has become depersonalized, some would even say "hardhearted". In most affluent countries, the number of family physicians and primary care doctors continues to decline. The trend towards highly specialized care works against a sympathetic doctor-patient relationship. In too many cases, the patient is no longer treated as a person, but rather as an assembly line of body parts each to be managed, often with great expertise, by an appropriate specialist.

In the views of at least some commentators, the rise of alternative medicine is a quest for more compassionate, personalized, and comprehensive health care. The trend is almost certainly also fuelled by a growing faith in so-called natural products as intrinsically good and safe, which is not at all a valid assumption. This faith is easy to exploit commercially.

It is less easy to exploit when traditional medicine is in the hands of properly trained, experienced, and licensed practitioners performing an ancient, culturally respected, and useful art of compassionate care and healing.

Ladies and gentlemen,

Last month, WHO issued its World Health Report, this year focused on primary health care and subtitled "Now more than ever". The report responds to calls made from all regions of the world for a renewal of primary health care.

Primary health care is a people-centred, holistic approach to health that makes prevention as important as cure. As part of this preventive approach, it tackles the root causes of ill health, also in non-health sectors, thus offering an upstream attack on threats to health.

Decades of experience tell us that primary health care produces better health outcomes, at lower costs, and with higher user satisfaction.

Let me stress this last point: higher user satisfaction. I personally find this one of the most striking findings in the report. As societies modernize, social expectations for health are rising all around the world. People want health care that is fair as well as efficient, comprehensive, and affordable. Studies show wide agreement. People surveyed in a range of countries believe that all members of society should have access to care and receive treatment when ill or injured, without going bankrupt as a result.

With this support from the World Health Report, my main conclusions should be obvious. I believe that the strong calls we are hearing for a renewal of primary health care create an ideal opportunity to revisit the place of traditional medicine, to take a positive look at its many contributions to health care that is equitable, accessible, affordable, and people-centred.

I believe this view is also captured in the draft Declaration of Beijing that you will be considering during this congress.

The two systems of traditional and Western medicine need not clash. Within the context of primary health care, they can blend together in a beneficial harmony, using the best features of each system, and compensating for certain weaknesses in each. This is not something that will happen all by itself. Deliberate policy decisions have to be made. But it can be done successfully.

Many countries have brought the two systems together in highly effective ways. In several countries where health systems are organized around primary health care, traditional medicine is well integrated and provides a backbone of much preventive care and treatment of common ailments.

Here in China, herbal therapy of proven utility in many disorders is provided in state hospitals throughout the country, alongside conventional medicine.

As I mentioned at the beginning, safeguards must be in place in the form of systems for regulation, training, and licensing or certification, and strict controls of product safety. Validation of the efficacy and safety of traditional medicines requires special research methodologies. WHO is providing support in this area, especially through the Special Programme for Research and Training in Tropical Diseases.

The time is also right to view traditional medicine as a precious resource. It needs to be respected and supported as a valuable source of leads for therapeutic advances and the discovery of new classes of drugs. I need mention only artemisinin for malaria to make this point.

Research and development in traditional medicine is part of the WHO global strategy and plan of action on public health, innovation and intellectual property adopted at this year's World Health Assembly. Apart from setting out a research agenda for traditional medicine, this action plan also addresses the need to prevent misappropriation of health-related traditional knowledge. WHO, together with the World Intellectual Property Organization, is also providing support in this area.

Ladies and gentlemen,

Public health owes the notion that prevention is better than cure to China and the *Huangdi Neijing*, the most important book of ancient Chinese medicine.

During its 3000-year history, traditional Chinese medicine

pioneered interventions such as diet, exercise, awareness of environmental influences on health, and the use of herbal remedies as part of a holistic approach to health.

Other ancient medical systems in other countries, such as Ayurveda in India, offer similar approaches to health. These are historical assets that have become all the more relevant given the three main ills of life in the 21st century: the globalization of unhealthy lifestyles, rapid unplanned urbanization, and demographic ageing. These are global trends with global consequences for health, most notably seen in the universal rise of chronic noncommunicable diseases, such as heart disease, cancer, diabetes, and mental disorders.

For these diseases and many other conditions, traditional medicine has much to offer in terms of prevention, comfort, compassion, and care.

This congress comes at an opportune time. The time has never been better, and the reasons never greater, for giving traditional medicine its proper place in addressing the many ills that face all our modern—and our traditional—societies.

Thank you.

(1799 words)

※ The text is extracted from the official website of WHO. https://www. who. int/dg/speeches/2008/20081107/en/

 Vocabulary

Ayurveda	[eɪɜː'viːdə]	n. 印度草医学
ailment	['eɪlmənt]	n. 病痛,疾病
malaria	[mə'leərɪə]	n. 疟疾
postpartum	[ˌpəʊst'pɑːtəm]	adj. 产后的
consensus	[kən'sensəs]	n. 共识,一致观点
obstetric	[əb'stetrɪk]	adj. 产科的
infrastructure	['ɪnfrəstrʌktʃə]	n. 基础设施
affluent	['æfluənt]	adj. 富裕的
orthodox	['ɔːθədɒks]	adj. 正统的,规范的
legitimate	[lɪ'dʒɪtɪmət]	adj. 合法的,合情合理的
surveillance	[sɜː'veɪləns]	n. 监督
rigorous	['rɪgərəs]	adj. 严格的,缜密的
intrinsically	[ɪn'trɪnzɪklɪ]	adv. 从本质上说

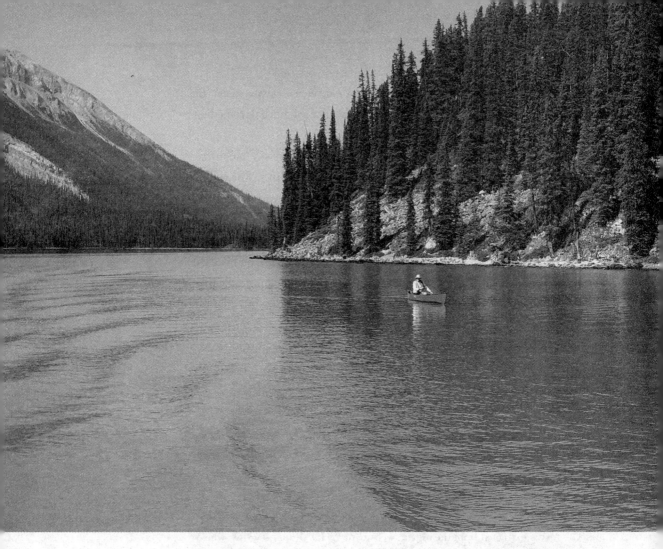

holistic	[həʊˈlɪstɪk]	*adj.* 整体的，全面的，功能整体性的
clash	[klæʃ]	*vi.* 碰撞，冲突
artemisinin	[ɑːtɪˈmiːsɪnɪn]	*n.* 青蒿素
demographic	[ˌdeməˈɡræfɪk]	*adj.* 人口统计的，人口统计学的
noncommunicable	[nɒnkəˈmjuːnɪkəbl]	*adj.* 非传染性的

◆ Questions

1. What is Dr Margaret Chan's attitude toward traditional medicine?

2. What do you think of traditional medicine? Is it a science or a witchcraft（巫术）?

3. In what way does traditional medicine help people's health?

4. Though faced with extremely strong doubt and disbelief, even severe crack-down from governments occasionally, traditional medicine still thrives and is in wide practice among patients, poor and rich alike. How come?

5. What should governments do with respect to traditional medicine?

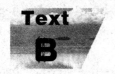

Address at Opening Ceremony of 9th Global Conference on Health Promotion

Li Keqiang
(*Premier of the State Council of the People's Republic of China*)

Dr Margaret Chan, Director-General of the WHO, distinguished guests, ladies and gentlemen, friends,

Good morning.

Health is a cornerstone for the comprehensive development and well-being of the people and a hallmark of national prosperity and social progress. On the occasion of the 9th Global Conference on Health Promotion, I wish to extend, on behalf of the Chinese government, warm congratulations on the opening of the conference and sincere welcome to all the distinguished guests.

This conference coincides with the 30th anniversary of the first International Conference on Health Promotion. Three decades ago, the Ottawa Charter introduced the concept of "health promotion", which has since guided the development of the health cause worldwide. Three decades on, thanks to the joint efforts of countries around the world and the hard work of the World Health Organization (WHO), the world average life expectancy has increased by over eight years. Maternal and infant mortality rate and that of children under five have been lowered by 50% on average, which is a big milestone in the history of human health.

At the same time, we should be aware that we are still confronted with daunting global health challenges. While traditional diseases, health issues and inequality in health remain acute, faster aging of the population, greater trans-border flows of people, the evolving spectrum of disease and changing environment and lifestyles are creating new problems. The threat of multiple diseases and our vulnerability to health risks have both risen. The sluggish world economic recovery and divergent trends of economic growth have added to the difficulty of ensuring the effective supply and the balanced and reasonable allocation of health resources. Promoting health remains an arduous task and nothing short of concerted international efforts is required for truly delivering the goal of "health for all".

This year marks the start of the implementation of the 2030 Agenda for Sustainable Development. The theme of this conference "health promotion in the sustainable development goals" highlights the important role of health promotion in global sustainable development endeavor. Discussions around this theme will go a long way to promoting consensus building and synergy for the full implementation of the Sustainable Development Goals (SDGs). In this connection, I would like to put forward the following suggestions.

—We should enhance policy dialogue and build a platform for health governance cooperation. Health promotion is the common endeavor of mankind. We should together build a community of shared future and take concrete actions to advance cooperation. We need to build a multilevel and wide-ranging institutional platform for dialogue and cooperation and support the WHO's efforts to lead, coordinate and implement global health programs. Efforts should also be made to improve health legislation in our respective countries and tighten regulation on health-impairing investment and trading activities through fiscal, taxation and financial policy tools.

At the same time, we need to uphold the principle of common but differentiated responsibilities and increase the representation and voice of developing countries. Developed countries should shoulder more responsibility and support developing countries. We should work together to make global health governance fairer and more reasonable.

—We should put in place an inclusive and interconnected system for prevention and control of global public health hazards. No country can stay immune to major public health challenges. Countries need to better coordinate health emergency practices, improve global mechanisms for disease surveillance, early-warning and emergency response, strengthen notification, information sharing and personnel training, and further improve global capacity to address public health emergencies. The Chinese government supports the WHO in putting together its global health emergency task force and contingency fund. We urge developed countries to step up support to developing countries in improving their public health systems, and together build up stronger lines of defense for global health.

—We should enhance the capacity for health supply and services through cooperation on innovation. Scientific and technological innovation is the golden key to health. Countries need to enhance research and development of health technologies, actively conduct bilateral and multilateral cooperation, including joint research on frontier and innovative technologies, and tackle common health hazards facing mankind together. We need to expand the network for exchange and cooperation in such areas as the prevention and control of antimicrobial resistance (AMR), advanced health technologies, drug research and development, energy-saving, emissions reduction and the treatment of pollution, and build platforms for entrepreneurship and innovation. There should be wider application and sharing of scientific and technological progress to bring greater benefits to more people.

—We should encourage mutual learning and promote greater integration between traditional and modern medical sciences. Throughout history, different countries and nations have developed their own views of health and acquired distinct strengths in the form of traditional medicine. Differences in medical practices should be embraced with equality and open-mindedness, and cultural exchanges be encouraged as a useful way to promote health cooperation. We should encourage mutual learning on the views and culture of health. We need to better promote traditional medicine, make better use of their strengths in preventing and treating diseases, and actively develop services trade in traditional medicine. By leveraging the complementarity between traditional and modern medical sciences, we will make new contribution to human health.

Ladies and Gentlemen, Friends,

China has been a strong advocate and firm practitioner of health promotion. Since the founding of the People's Republic, in particular since reform and opening-up, China has vigorously expanded health care services despite a relatively underdeveloped economy. We have significantly improved the health of our people, and found a path of health development consistent with China's national conditions. In 2009, China started a new round of health care reform. We identified a core objective, which is to offer basic health care services to all people as a public good, and outlined the principle of ensuring basic levels of health care, strengthening community health services and building up health care networks.

Important progress has been made in this direction. We put in place a system of basic medical insurance that covers the entire population of over 1.3 billion people, offering institutional guarantee for universal access. We improved basic rural health service network at county, township and village levels and the system of urban community health services, making such services more convenient and accessible for our people. We took vigorous measures to promote equal access to public health services and offered basic public health services for all urban and rural residents for free. Our spending on public health services has been growing year by year and will continue to grow. We worked out a Chinese solution to advance health care reform, which is a world-wide challenge.

China's average life expectancy now stands at 76.3 years. Maternal mortality rate was reduced to 20.1 per 100,000 and infant mortality rate 8.1 per 1,000, generally better than the average level in middle and high income countries. For the largest developing country with over 1.3 billion people, such accomplishments are no mean feat.

China is at a decisive stage for building a moderately prosperous society in all respects. At the recently held National Health Conference, the first in the new century, President Xi Jinping outlined in an important speech the overall guidelines, targets and tasks for building a healthy China from a strategic and overarching perspective and proposed principles for health-related work. We will focus on the grassroots, pursue reform and innovation as a driving force and disease prevention as the priority, give importance to both traditional Chinese medicine and western medicine, incorporate health into all policy-making, and strive for participation by all and benefits to all. We promulgated the Outline of Healthy China 2030 Plan with the aim to provide all-dimensional, whole-of-the-life-cycle health services for all by 2030, increase average life expectancy to 79 years, and reach high-income countries' level in main health indicators. With this in mind, we will make relentless efforts in the following areas:

—We will take health as a strategic priority to advance health in tandem with economic and social progress. We will prioritize health in development planning, highlight health targets in economic and social programs, give more weight to health in drafting and implementing public policies, and meet health demand in fiscal spending, with a view to providing basic health services for all.

—We will build a whole-process health promotion system to protect people's health throughout the life cycle. There are many factors affecting people's health from the beginning to the end of life. We need to provide whole-of-the-life-cycle health services for the people. Effective measures will be taken for prevention, health care and greater intervention to make people healthier and less vulnerable. We will enhance health education, spread health knowledge and skills, deepen fitness campaigns for all, raise people's health awareness and sense of responsibility, and foster a new health system in which all people will participate, contribute and benefit. We will strengthen prevention and control of major diseases, improve prevention and treatment practices, enforce cross-agency holistic measures at all levels, and reduce damage on people's health from major diseases. We will intensify pollution treatment and foster a sound environment for people's health.

—We will work hard to improve community-level health care and strengthen weak links to increase fairness and accessibility of health services. The biggest weak link in China's health system lies at the community level, in rural and poor areas in particular. We will coordinate urban and rural development and pursue a new type of urbanization, make more resources available for community-level health programs. Communities must be equipped with greater capacity of disease prevention and control through cultivating general physicians and providing long-distance medical treatment and paired-up assistance. The advantages of traditional Chinese medicine must be harnessed to widen the availability of medical care and health services. We will implement health-related poverty-alleviation programs, intensify support for poor areas in insurance for major diseases and medical assistance, prevent disease-induced poverty, and narrow the gap in basic health services between urban and rural areas and among different regions and groups of people.

—We will continue to deepen health care reform and set up basic health care systems that cover urban and rural areas. Our reform in this area is now in a deep-water zone, which calls for greater courage and wisdom. We will further deepen public hospital reform, quicken the development of tiered medical services, cut red tapes and enhance coordination among medical and health care institutions at various levels and of different categories. This way, we hope to provide high-quality medical services to our people, and help community-level medical institutions improve their performance. Progress has been made in encouraging big, medium-sized and small hospitals and township hospitals to establish the Health Care Alliance (HCA), which would make medical services more accessible and affordable for the people.

——We will build up a nationwide basic medical insurance system, reform the way of making medical insurance payouts, merge the basic medical insurance systems for rural and non-working urban residents, and establish a nationwide information network for medical insurances to improve quality and efficiency. We will also reform the supply system of pharmaceuticals to deliver safe and effective medicine to our people. We will advance coordinated reform of medical services, medical insurance and the medicine industry, motivate medical practitioners, including by making their jobs even more dignified, and enhance the vitality and sustainability of medical and health care systems.

——We will vigorously develop the health sector to better meet people's increasingly diverse health needs. With higher standards of living and greater awareness about health, our people expect more multi-tiered, diversified and individualized products and services. To respond to their demands, government and market both have a role to play. The government needs to ensure basic supply, especially for the most vulnerable groups, while the market can be more active in providing non-basic and more diversified health services. We will encourage increased supply of health products and services from non-governmental sources, and the setting-up of privately run hospitals, thus making it easier for people to get more affordable medical treatment. We will support innovation in medical science and boost integrated development between the health sector and old-age care, tourism, the Internet, fitness and recreation and food industries. We will also promote mass innovation and entrepreneurship in the health sector and practice the "Internet Plus Health" action plan, so that new industries, new businesses and new models will thrive in this sector.

China has been actively calling for and contributing to global health cooperation, and has fulfilled its due international

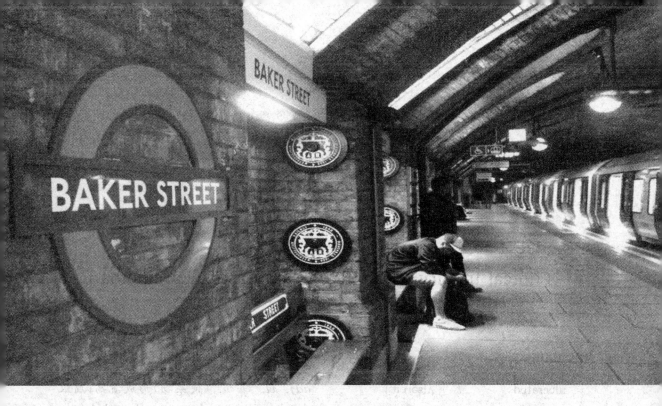

responsibilities and obligations. During the past half a century, China has sent over 20,000 medical staff to 67 countries and regions, treating patients for over 260 million times. China has contributed its share to the fight against the Ebola epidemic that broke out in West Africa in 2014. China moved promptly to dispatch over 1,200 medical staff and public health experts, who fought against the disease side by side with the people in the affected countries. China highly appreciates the prominent role that the WHO has played over the years in curbing communicable diseases and coordinating global health affairs. Under the framework of the UN and the WHO, China will continue to actively participate in global health promotion efforts and do its best to provide assistance to other developing countries.

Ladies and Gentlemen, Friends,

Health is an eternal pursuit of mankind, and health promotion is the shared responsibility of the international community. Let us work together to make our world a better and healthier place!

In conclusion, I wish this conference full success.

Thank you.

(2254 words)

※ The text is extracted from the official website of the State Council of the People's Republic of China. http://english. gov. cn/premier/speeches/2016/11/23/content - 281475498309138. htm

Practice 1

Clinical Inquiry—Case Report on Gastric Carcinoma

 Vocabulary

ulcerated	[ˈʌlsəreɪt]	*adj. vt.* & *vi.* (使某物)形成溃疡；腐败 develop into or become affected by an ulcer
intermittent	[ˌɪntəˈmɪtənt]	*adj.* 间歇的；断断续续的 occurring at irregular intervals; not continuous or steady
abdominal ultrasound	[æbˈdɒmɪnl ˈʌltrəsaʊnd]	腹部超声 the ultrasonic used in medical imaging on the belly
pylori	[paɪˈlɔːraɪ]	*n.* 幽门，幽门部 (pylorus 的名词复数) the opening from the stomach into the duodenum (small intestine)
peptic ulcer	[ˌpeptɪk ˈʌlsə]	*n.* 胃溃疡 a lesion in the lining (mucosa) of the digestive tract, typically in the stomach or duodenum, caused by the digestive action of pepsin and stomach acid
endoscopy	[enˈdɒskəpɪ]	*n.* 内镜检查术 a medical examination of a hollow organ of the body
diabetes mellitus	[ˌdaɪəˈbiːtiːz ˈmɪlɪəs]	糖尿病；……型糖尿病
hypertension	[ˌhaɪpəˈtenʃn]	*n.* 高血压 a medical condition in which the blood pressure is extremely high
lipid	[ˈlɪpɪd]	*n.* 脂类 the lipids are a large and diverse group of naturally occurring organic compounds that are related by their solubility in nonpolar organic solvents

		(e. g. ether, chloroform, acetone & benzene） and general insolubility in water
gastroesophageal reflux disease(GERD)		胃食管返流疾病
diverticulosis	[ɑɪvətɪkjuˈləʊsɪs]	*n.*（肠）憩室病 a condition in which diverticula are present in the intestine without signs of inflammation
osteopenia	[ɒstiːəʊˈpiːnɪə]	*n.* 骨质减少 reduced bone mass of lesser severity than osteoporosis
adenocarcinoma	[ˌædnəʊˌkɑːsəˈnəʊmə]	*n.* 腺癌 a malignant tumor formed from glandular structures in epithelial tissue
epigastric	[ˌepɪˈgæstrɪk]	上腹部疼痛

Using Lay Terms in Explanations

Explanations should be given in words the patients will understand, avoiding medical terms. Using lay terms—words familiar to people without medical knowledge—can help patients understand explanations. e. g. :

Medical Terms	Lay Terms
1. intermittent	not continuous
2. epigastric	the upper middle region of the abdomen

Sample Dialogue

(chief complaint, history of present illness, history of past illness, personal history, physical exam medical examination)

Case Report on Gastric Carcinoma: At the Office of Oncology Department

Chief: Morning, everyone, now let's begin today's work.

Intern: August 21st, 2017, morning. Total number of the patients is 28, including 1 new admission, no critical patients, and all the patients are in stable condition.

Chief: I'm glad to know the patients are all in stable condition. Now Doctor Wei, could you give us a case report of the newly patient.

Doctor Wei: All right. The newly patient in Bed 16 is Mrs. Wu, female, 69 years old.

Chief complaint: Ulcerated tumor in the body of the stomach.

History of present illness: The patient presented to the physician with a four-week history of intermittent chest pressure radiating to her back. Extensive evaluation for a cardiac source was unremarkable, including a normal stress test and abdominal ultrasound. She then developed epigastric abdominal pain, and given that she carried a history of prior H. pylori infection in 2003, there was a concern that she might have a peptic ulcer. An upper endoscopy was obtained and showed a large ulcerated tumor in the body of the stomach.

History of past illness: Type II diabetes mellitus, hypertension, elevated lipids, gastroesophageal reflux disease(GERD), diverticulosis, endometriosis, kidney stones, anxiety and osteopenia.

Personal history: She never smoked and did not drink alcohol.

Family history: No family history of stomach cancer, but her older brother died of colon cancer metastatic to the liver and lung at the age of 80.

Physical exam: T: 36.2　P: 90bpm　R: 18/min　BP: 182/90mmHg

Chief: What about her pathological examination?

Doctor Wei: Pathological examination of biopsy specimens of the stomach ulcer showed moderately to poorly differentiated adenocarcinoma. Staging computed tomography (CT) scans of the chest, abdomen and pelvis only showed prominent lymph nodes adjacent to the lesser curvature of the stomach within the gastrohepatic ligament and no evidence of metastatic disease.

There was mild epigastric tenderness without a palpable massor an enlarged liver. results of a complete blood count, plasma levels of electrolytes and tests of kidney and liver function were normal.

Chief: Thank you, Doctor Wei.

Activities and Role-play (inviting students to improvise and act it out)

Practice 2

International Conference
—Opening Remarks and Introducing Lecturers

 Useful Expressions of Presiders' Opening Remarks

1. Distinguished guests, Ladies and gentlemen, good morning/afternoon! On behalf

of Dr. Hank Bakedam, the World Health Organization Representative in China, I would like to thank the organizers for holding this very important and timely discussion on Depression and Suicide in the Elderly.

2. Excellency, Mr. Prime Minister/Excellencies, Ladies and Gentlemen, Dear Friends, we are gathered here for the worthiest of human purposes—to save the lives and improve the health and well-being of the world's most vulnerable children and women.

3. Respected/Honorable Delegates and Members of this Association (Organization, Union...), on behalf of UNICEF and the larger UN family committed to "Deliver as One", I would like to extend our full solidarity and support for National Partnership for Maternal, Newborn and Child Health.

4. Good morning/afternoon/evening! Dear Friends/Colleagues/Confreres, Milton Dance Head and Neck Center at the Great Baltimore Medical Center was established to honor Milton Lady Dance's 25-year head and neck cancer survivor,... Now I'd like to introduce Dr. Joseph coming into the director to introduce the 2012 Milton Dance lecture.

 ## Useful Expressions for Introducing Lecturers/Speakers

1. We are very fortunate to have Dr. X as our guest speaker this afternoon. I would like to give a brief account of the excellent work which he has done in connection with ... during last five years. The title of Dr. X's lecture today is ... We look forward to a stimulating talk from him in this very interesting subject, and it's a great pleasure to call on him now to give his lecture.

2. I have great pleasure of introducing Professor Edward from University of London, He has kindly agreed to address us on the subject of ...

3. Mr. Cart is a distinguished professor from the United States. He is going to talk about ...

4. It gives me great pleasure to introduce our guest speaker today. Dr. X is a professor of chemistry at University of X. His main research interest is in ... and he is a distinguished investigator in his important filed. This morning he is going to tell us about ... Dr. X, please.

5. We are greatly privileged to have Professor Cart on my left. He has kindly agreed to address us on the subject of ...

6. The next special lecture is being presented by Dr. Bench, Professor of Medicine at London University. We feel grateful that he has taken time from his busy schedule to spend this hour with us. Dr. Bench's research interests in ... was initially inspired by his first professor, Dr. Cooper, who you know well, and Dr. Bench has been very active in this important field ever since. Today he will be talking to

us about ... I am sure his address will be well worth your attention. Dr. Bench, please!

7. And our next lecturer helps with that because the surgeons when we made the road possible for any types of vehicles, he fixes that problem, repairs the road, and sometimes he makes it even better than it was. So Doctor Fu-Chan Wei is truly a giant in his field. He became Chairman of public plastic reconstruction surgery, Chang Gung Memorial Hospital in Taiwan. He made very similar contribution to the development of free tissue transfer reconstruction including the fibular free flap ... So I don't want to take more time, and let's welcome him and look forward to his talk.

Useful Expressions for Self-introduction

1. Thank you very much for your instruction, and John and Joe. Good morning, my friends. Ladies and Gentlemen, it's an indeed great pleasure and honor for me to speak to you in this very important occasion. I'm going to share with you my thoughts and my approach of segmental mandibular defect reconstruction.

2. Let me introduce myself. My name is ... from ... Institute. It is a privilege for me to give my speech.

3. I am honored and proud to address here to you distinguished audience of the 8th International Conference on gastric cancer here in Paris.

4. It is a personal privilege for me to be here in Paris as a lecturer for this International Conference on ... I'm from the Chemical Physics Department of Oxford University. I'll speak on ...

 Activities and Role-play (inviting students to improvise and act it out)

Practice 3

Oral English for Culture and on Social Occasions
—Basic Understanding of a City

Occasion: Basic Understanding of a City around the City Construction, Transportation and Climate

Useful Expressions for City Construction，Transportation and Climate

City Construction

urban 都市的

suburban 郊区的

urbanization 城市化

resource of drinking water 饮用水源

forestation coverage in the city 城市绿化覆盖

housing accumulation funds 住房公积金

matched public installations 配套的公共设施

satellite city 卫星城

overpass 立交桥

central heating 集中供热

power plant 发电站

substation 变电站

transmission line 输电线路

garden city 园林城市

waterworks 水厂

sewage treatment plant 污水处理厂

gas/liquefied petroleum gas and natural gas 煤气/液化石油和天然气

Transportation

air traffic hub 空中交通枢纽

railway station 火车站

passenger ferry terminal 客运码头

public transportation 公共交通枢纽

interchange 轨道交通枢纽

tourist bus center 旅游集散中心

BRT(Bus Rapid Transit) 快速公交

double deck buses 双层公交

long-distance bus 长途汽车

metro 轨道交通(地铁、轻轨)

maglev train 磁悬浮列车

taxi 出租车

wharf 货运码头

Climate/weather

weather forecast 天气预报

sandstorm 沙尘暴

thunderstorm 雷雨

typhoon 台风

moderate snow 中雪

fog 雾

sleet 雨夹雪

overcast 阴天

frost 霜冻

snowy 有雪的

drizzle 毛毛雨

monsoon 季风

rainy season (梅)雨季节

tropical high 热带高压

greenhouse effect 温室效应

heat island effect 热岛效应

warm in winter and cool in summer 冬暖夏凉

Sample Sentences

1. The urban area is the center of the development of society and economy.
2. The garden city attracts many tourists.
3. Can I reach the park by metro?
4. Bus Rapid Transit，also called BRT，is a new model of public transportation.

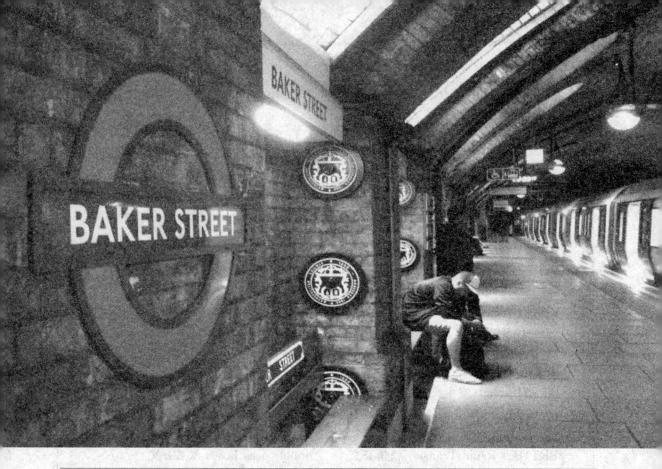

5. You will be required to leave a deposit when you pick up the car.

6. These seats are meant for elderly and handicapped persons and women with child.

7. When the bus is moving, do not speak to the driver.

8. Is this the right counter to check in for my flight?

9. Where can we take a shuttle bus?

10. Could you tell me where I can find the taxi to go to Terminal 6?

11. Excuse me, which bus should I take to railway station?

12. The sharing-bike, a new way of green transport, provides people an alternative to get a short-distance site instead of walking or taking a taxi.

13. I don't think the rain could last long.

14. What's the average temperature in Hefei on a summer's day?

15. Is the weather always like this?

16. It's clearing up.

17. I'm so sorry it has turned out wet.

18. I hope the weather stays this way.

19. The weather forecast says it will be cloudy tomorrow.

20. I think the snow is going to last all day.

Topics for Further Discussion

1. The characteristics and styles of different cities in China
2. The development of transport in China over the past few decades
3. The climate differences between north and south of China

References for Further Discussion

1. Beijing is famous for its ancient architectures, such as the Forbidden City, the Temple of Heaven, the Great Wall, the Summer Palace, the Temple of Heaven, etc. Also, Beijing has impressive modern architectures, such as Water Cube, Bird's Nest, National Grand Theater, and China Central Television Headquarters. The combination and contrast of ancient architectures with post-modern architectures represent Beijing's past and future.

   Western architectural buildings, such as the Bund, and Pudong super skyscrapers are on behalf of Shanghai's architectural features. The charm of these buildings, lies in not only its long history, but also its Western, Oriental and modern styles. I think it is the charm and the city mark of Shanghai.

   Suzhou gardens have a long history, more than 200 gardens throughout the ancient city in the Song, Yuan, Ming and Qing dynasties. The classical gardens of Suzhou are masterpieces of Chinese landscape garden design in which art, nature, and ideas are integrated perfectly to create ensembles of great beauty and peaceful harmony. The most famous gardens are: the Lion Park, Lingering Garden, and Humble Administrator's Garden.

2. Transport in China has experienced major growth and expansion in recent years. Much of contemporary China's transport systems have been built since the establishment of the People's Republic of China in 1949. The railway, which is the primary mode of long distance transport, has seen rapid growth reaching 120,970 km of railway lines making it the second longest network in the world. Prior to 1950, there were only 21,800 km of railway lines. The extensive rail network includes the longest and busiest HSR network in the world with 19,000 km of high-speed lines. While rail travel remains the most popular form of intercity transport, air travel has also experienced significant growth since the late 1990s. Major airports such as Beijing Capital International Airport and Shanghai Pudong International Airport are among the busiest ones in the world. At the end of 2016, there are some 30 metro systems in operation across China, including some of the largest and busiest subway networks in the world. Additionally, many bus rapid transits, light rail and rapid transit lines are currently under construction or in the planning stages across the country. The highway and road systems also have gone through rapid expansion, resulting in a rapid increase of motor vehicle use

throughout China.

3. China has always had an undefined border between its Northern and Southern regions. The eastern provinces, such as Jiangsu and Anhui perceive the Yangtze River as the dividing line between the two main parts of China, but the more ancient geographical dividing line is still the so-called Huai River-Qinling Mountains line in the middle of the given country.

China's climate is divided into six categories as follows: tropical, subtropical, warm-temperate, temperate, cold-temperate, and Qinghai-Tibet Plateau temperate zone. Most of the country lies in the northern temperate zone, which is characterized by warm climate and well-defined seasons, being suitable for habitation. Actually, the climate in China varies greatly from south to north, especially in winter when dry and cold winds, blowing from Siberia and the Mongolian Plateau, lead to a huge temperature gap between south (above 0 ℃) and north (far below 0 ℃) China. In summers, however, except for a few remote places, there is little temperature difference between Northern and Southern China for there are overall high temperatures in almost the whole country.

Unit 5

Key Points

Learning Targets
- To master the skill of *retelling*
- To learn the skill of *paraphrasing*
- To learn about the academic terms of pediatrics in clinical diagnostic conversation

Learning Focus
- How to declare the theme and make requirements to the audience at an international academic conference

Cultural Points
- Traditional Chinese art

✓音、视频资源
✓参考译文
✓参考答案
✓学术探讨

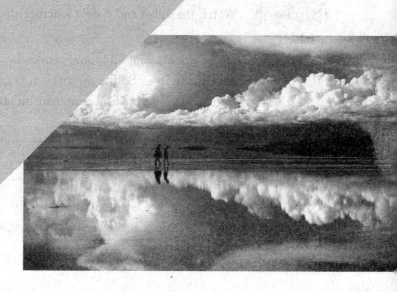

Video 1

A Clinical Research about the Influence
of Protandim on Cancer

Exercise Ⅰ   Watch the video and fill in the blanks.

It has been a ___1___ for a number of years. Is anti-oxidative ___2___ a good idea here? Because you may actually ___3___ the cells that you want to kill, using an therapy that puts focus ___4___ stress on the cells, with the idea of pushing them over the ___5___ , killing them. And therefore, I've recommended to everyone who's asked me for the last five years "Should I take Protandim if I got a cancer ___6___ , I am about to undergo ___7___ or ___8___ ." And my conservative response has been, because this is controversial. Some scientists argue "Don't do it, because you may protect the cancer"; other experts say "Do it, because you may protect the other ___9___ more than you protect the cancer." We didn't really have a ___10___ answer.

Exercise Ⅱ   Watch the video and decide whether the following statements are true (T) or false (F).

11. Protandim is greatly amplified and works better than curcumin because we get this energy of the five. So the mechanism is quite different.

12. Akor Ward works in a medical center in India, well known in the field of NRF2 activators.

13. Tumors are treated with chemotherapy and with radiation. The reason for treating tumors with those two treatments is that they both decrease oxidative stress substantially.

14. Anti-oxidative therapy is a good idea, because it damages the cancer cells only.

15. Activating NRF2 has a bigger effect, because it sensitizes the tumors to radiation and chemo.

Yoav Medan: Ultrasonic Surgery-Noninvasive Healing

Exercise I   Watch the video and fill in the blanks of the following.

So the first one is in the __1__. One of the neurological conditions that can be treated with __2__ is movement disorder, like Parkinson's or essential tremor. What is typical to those conditions, for __3__ for example is inability to drink or eat cereal or soup without __4__ everything all over you, or write legibly so people can understand it, and be really __5__ in your life without the help of others.

So I'd like you to meet John. John is a retired professor of history from Virginia. So he __6__ essential tremor for many years. And __7__ didn't help him anymore. And many of those patients refused to undergo __8__ to have people cut into their brain. And about four or five months ago, he __9__ an experimental procedure. It is approved under an FDAIDE at the University of Virginia in Charlottesville, using focused ultrasound to __10__ a point in his thalamus.

Exercise II   Watch the video and decide whether the following statements are true (T) or false (F).

11. When a physician takes a regular MRI scan on patients, different organs will be attached by the same transducer.
12. The area around the target in the thalamus is dangerous.
13. When the physician takes a regular MRI scan, the only device he needs to use is a mouse.
14. The first sonication will elevate the temperature by a few degrees, so it will be at higher energy, and may cause some damage.
15. During the ablation, the physician must manage the accurate time-control, or it will basically destroy the proteins of the cells.

Listening 1 ▌▌▌▌

Accelerate Expansion of Antiretroviral Therapy to All People Living with HIV: WHO

Exercise 丨   Choose one correct answer from A, B, C, and D.

1. What is the key to end the AIDS epidemic within a generation?
   A. Expanding the traditional therapy to people with HIV
   B. Further expanding the science development
   C. Further expanding antiretroviral therapy
   D. Expanding the retroviral therapy

2. What's the peak time of AIDS epidemic?
   A. 2004   B. 2015   C. 2020   D. 2030

3. Which place is more likely to provide treatment for its people with HIV?
   A. In Africa   B. In America   C. In Asia   D. In Australia

4. People living with HIV are more likely to _____, if they begin antiretroviral therapy soon after acquiring the virus.
   A. damage your immune system
   B. more likely to transmit the virus to their partners
   C. stay healthy
   D. above A, B, C

5. WHO is now presenting an additional set of recommendations on how to expand ART to all of the following except _____.
   A. using innovative testing approaches
   B. starting treatment faster in those people who are diagnosed with HIV
   C. bringing ART to the community
   D. abandoning clinic visits for people who have been stable on ART for some time

医学英语学术交流教程

Listening 2

Kidney Calculus

 Vocabulary

crystallize	['krɪstəˌlaɪz]	v. 使结晶；使成形
oxalate	['ɒksəˌleɪt]	n. 草酸盐
phosphate	['fɒsfeɪt]	n. 磷酸盐
magnesium	[mæg'niːzɪəm]	n. 镁
ammonium	[ə'məʊnɪəm]	n. 铵
magnesium ammonium phosphate (＝struvite)		n. 磷酸铵镁
excruciating	[ɪk'skruːʃɪeɪtɪŋ]	adj. 极度的，使苦恼的
alpha blockers		甲型肾上腺素阻断剂
potassium citrate		柠檬酸钾
pulverize	['pʌlvəraɪz]	v. 粉碎
extracorporeal	[ˌekstrəkɔː'pɔːrɪəl]	adj. 身体外的
lithotripsy	['laɪθəʊtrɪpsɪ]	n. （肾结石等）震波碎石
incision	[ɪn'sɪʒn]	n. 切开，切口
groin	[grɒɪn]	n. 腹股沟
rhubarb	['ruːbɑːb]	n. 大黄

Exercise Ⅰ Crossword the following words based on what you've listened. You may refer to the hints in the Across-Down region below if necessary.

jostle	stent	groin	dilute
tract	clump	calculus	address
incision	zap		

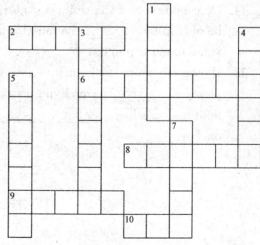

ACROSS	DOWN
2 the part of the body where the legs join at the top including the area around the genitals (=sex organs)	1 a system of connected organs or tissues along which materials or messages pass
6 a hard lump produced by the concretion of mineral salts; found in hollow organs or ducts of the body	3 a sharp cut made in sth, particularly during a medical operation; the act of making a cut in sth
8 to make a liquid weaker by adding water or another liquid to it	4 to push roughly against sb in a crowd
9 a small support that is put inside a blood or other vessel tube in the body, for example in order to stop sth blocking it	5 to think about a problem or a situation and decide how you are going to deal with it
10 to destroy, kill or hit sb/sth suddenly and with force, esp. by remote-controlling	7 a small group of things or people very close together, especially particles, trees or plants

Exercise II Fill in the blanks with the original words and phrases or with expressions which have the same or the closest meaning.

11. The renal calculus which on record was more than _____ is the biggest kidney stone and it weighed more than a kilogram.

12. It's common for surgeons to detect a kidney stone, which is a hard mass of crystals, forming in the part of _____, _____, _____ or your urethra in human bodies.

13. A stone's travelling through a kidney and into the ureter can be accompanied by symptoms of _____, _____ and _____ while urinating.

14. On condition that the stone is slightly larger, medications like alpha blockers can be of help by _____ the muscles in the ureter and making it _____ for the stone to get through.

15. If you are prone to kidney stone, you're now strongly recommended drinking plenty of _____, which dilutes the calcium oxalate and other compounds and limiting foods like _____, _____, _____, and rhubarb which are high in oxalate.

Part II Reading Comprehension

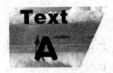

Text A

The Prevention of Infection-Associated Cancers

Silvio De Flora & Paolo Bonanni

Collectively, chronic viral and bacterial infections and trematode infestations have been estimated to be associated with approximately one of five human cancers worldwide. The fraction attributable to each one of the chronic infections caused by hepatitis B and C viruses (HBV and HCV), human papilloma viruses (HPV) and helicobacter pylori is about 5%. These infections are the most important causes of major types of cancer, including hepatocellular carcinoma, cervical cancer and stomach cancer, respectively. Taking into account the mechanisms of infection-related carcinogenesis, integrated approaches are addressed to the control of the associated infection as well as to avoidance of cancer occurrence and progression. Large-scale interventions have been implemented, such as the anti-HBV and anti-HPV routine vaccination programs. The latter has been designed with the specific goal of preventing HPV-associated cancers, which is an outstanding breakthrough in cancer prevention. Intriguingly, not only prevention but even therapy of an infectious disease and eradication of a pathogen become a crucial tool for the primary prevention of these cancers.

Overview of microbial and parasitic diseases associated with human cancers

While the discovery that viruses can cause tumors in animals traces back to one century ago, the implication of microbial and parasitic diseases in the causation of human cancers has been demonstrated more recently. The burden of infection-associated cancers depends on a variety of factors. An important one is the geographic area, since certain chronic viral and bacterial infections and trematode infestations have a greater epidemiological impact in developing countries, as compared with developed countries, where only 16% of the world population resides. This circumstance is due to the higher endemicity, in developing countries, of infectious and parasitic diseases posing carcinogenic risks and to the lower availability of both preventive and therapeutic tools aimed at curing the disease or at avoiding its chronic evolution.

The proportions of cancer deaths attributable to viral and bacterial infections and to parasitic diseases were estimated by Doll et al. to be 10% in the USA in 1981 and by Doll to be 10%—20% in UK in 1998. Pisani et al. estimated that 15.6% (1,450,000 cases) of the worldwide incidence of cancers in 1990 could be attributed either to hepatitis B virus (HBV), hepatitis C virus (HCV), human papillomavirus (HPV), Epstein-Barr virus, human T-cell lymphothropic (T-cell leukaemia/lymphoma) virus (HTLV)-1, human immunodeficiency virus (HIV), Helicobacter pylori, schistosomes or liver flukes. These data were updated in 2006 by Parkin who, based on the evidence of the strength of association and the prevalence of infection in different geographic areas, estimated that the total infection-attributable cancer in the year 2002 was 1.9 million cases, which accounted for 17.8% of all cancers in the world. By preventing cancer-associated infectious diseases, there would be 26.3% fewer cases in developing countries (<1.5 million cases/year) and 7.7% fewer cases in developed countries (<390,000 cases). In 2009, zur Hausen estimated that slightly >20% of the global cancer burden can be linked to infectious agents and predicted that this fraction will increase in the future.

The infections with HBV and HCV, which are the only hepatitis virus infections that tend to evolve chronically, are associated with occurrence of hepatocellular carcinoma (HCC). HBV and HCV infections were estimated to be associated with 4.9% of all cancer cases and specifically with 85.5% of all HCC cases in the world, 54.4% of which attributable to HBV and 31.1% attributable to HCV according to Parkin. A similar figure (80.0%) was confirmed by zur Hausen. Liver cancer is the third leading cause of cancer death in men and the sixth among women, with an expected number of 680,000 deaths in 2007.

Papillomaviruses and polyomaviruses are DNA viruses that formerly belonged to the family of papovaviridae, together with simian virus 40 (SV40) or vacuolizing virus. In fact, the papova prefix combines the two initial letters of papilloma, polioma and vacuolizing. HPV infections were estimated to account for 5.2% of all cancers in the world, being responsible for 3% of mouth cancers, 12% of oropharynx cancers, 40% of penis cancers, 40% of vulva/vagina cancers and virtually 100% of uterine cervix cancers. Cervical cancer is the second most commonly diagnosed cancer in women and is the third leading cause of cancer death in women worldwide. An estimated 309,800 deaths were expected to occur in 2007, more than 83% of which in developing countries.

Several bacteria are known or suspected to be related to cancers in humans. The most important is H. pylori, formerly named Campylobacter pyloridis or C. pylori, a spiral or slightly curved gram-negative bacterium with two to six characteristic unipolar flagella, which is the main cause of chronic gastritis in humans and has been associated with both gastric cancer and gastric B-cell mucosa-associated lymphoid tissue lymphoma (MALT). Helicobacter pylori was estimated to be associated with 5.5% of all cancers and specifically with 63.4% or 80.0% of stomach cancers. Note that stomach cancer, in 2007, was expected to remain the fourth most common malignancy in the world, with 1 million new cases, 70% of which in developing countries.

Of other possible bacteria related to cancer, Streptococcus bovis is a normal inhabitant of the human gastrointestinal tract that, according to several studies, may be involved in colorectal carcinogenesis. Chronic infection of the gallbladder with Salmonella typhi increases the risk of developing gallbladder carcinoma. Arthropod-borne bartonellae cause persistent infection of erythrocytes and endothelial cells, whose massive proliferation can lead to vascular tumor formation in humans. Besides exogenous bacteria, it has been suspected that indigenous microbes may play a role in cancer risk because they are part of our metabolism and makeup. The human gut microbiome has been implicated in the etiology of localized intestinal diseases such as the irritable bowel syndrome, inflammatory bowel disease and colon cancer. In addition, there is epidemiological evidence that the obligate intracellular Chlamydophila (formerly Chlamydia) pneumoniae may be associated with chronic lung diseases, also including lung cancer.

In addition, infestations with trematode worms belonging to the phylum Platyhelminthes have been associated with human cancers.

The association of Schistosoma haematobium infestation with urinary bladder cancer is well established, whereas infestation with Schistosoma japonicum is possibly associated with colorectal cancer and liver cancer. Both colorectal viverrini and chlonorchis sinensis infestations convincingly demonstrated to be associated with occurrence of cholangiocarcinoma.

Thus, on the whole, it appears that persistent infections are the leading causes for some of the most important human cancers, such as stomach cancer, cervical cancer and liver cancer. Collectively, their impact on human cancer epidemiology is just lower than that of the two dominating, lifestyle-related causes of cancer, i. e. tobacco smoking and dietary factors. Individually, the risk attributable to each one of the three major viral (HPV, HBV/HCV) and bacterial (H. pylori) chronic infections is higher than that attributable to important risk factors, such as environmental pollution.

(1191 words)

※ The text is extracted from *Advance Access Publication*, March 24, 2011.

Vocabulary

trematode	['tremətəud]	n. & adj. 吸虫(的)
papillomavirus	[pæpɪləu'mævaɪrəs]	n. 乳头瘤病毒属
helicobacter	[helɪ'kɒbæktə]	n. 螺杆菌
hepatocellular	[hepətəu'seljulə]	adj. 肝细胞的
carcinoma	[ˌkɑːsɪ'nəumə]	n. 癌
cervical	['səːvɪkl]	adj. [解]颈的;子宫颈的
carcinogenesis	[kɑːsɪnəu'dʒenɪsɪs]	n. 癌病变,致癌作用
eradication	[ɪˌrædɪ'keɪʃn]	n. 摧毁,根除
parasitic	[ˌpærə'sɪtɪk]	adj. 寄生(物)的;由寄生虫引起的
epidemiological	[ˌepɪˌdiːmɪə'lɒdʒɪkl]	adj. 流行病学的
endemicity	[endɪ'mɪsɪtɪ]	n. 地方的特性,风土性
therapeutic	[ˌθerə'pjuːtɪkəl]	adj. 治疗(学)的
Epstein-Barr virus (EBV)	['epstaɪn baːr]	EB 病毒
schistosome	['ʃɪstəˌsəum]	n. 血吸虫,裂体吸虫
fluke	[fluk]	n. 吸虫,蛭
polyomavirus	[pəuljəu'mævaɪrəs]	n. 多瘤病毒
vacuolizing	[vækjuəulaɪzɪŋ]	adj. 空泡的
oropharynx	[əurə'færɪŋks]	n. 口咽
penis	['piːnɪs]	n. 阴茎

vulva	[ˈvʌlvə]	n. 阴户
vagina	[vəˈdʒaɪnə]	n. 阴道
gastric	[ˈgæstrɪk]	adj. 胃的；胃部的
mucosa	[mjuːˈkəʊsə]	n. 黏膜
streptococcus bovis	[ˌstreptəˈkɒkəs] [bɒvɪs]	n. 牛链球菌
colorectal	[kəʊləˈrektəl]	adj. 结肠直肠的
gallbladder	[ˈgɔːlˌblædə]	n. 胆囊
arthropod-borne	[ˈɑːθrəpɒdˈbɔːn]	虫媒传播
bartonella	[ˌbɑːtəˈnelə]	n. 巴尔通氏体属
erythrocyte	[ɪˈrɪθrəsaɪt]	n. 红细胞；红血球
endothelial	[ˌendəˈθiːlɪəl]	adj. 内皮的
exogenous	[ekˈsɒdʒənəs]	adj. 外生的，外成的，外因的
indigenous	[ɪnˈdɪdʒənəs]	adj. 自身固有的，内因的
gut	[gʌt]	n. 勇气；内脏；直觉；肠
etiology	[ˌiːtɪˈɒlədʒɪ]	n. 病因学，病源论
intestinal	[ˌɪntesˈtaɪnl]	adj. 肠的；肠壁；肠道细菌
bowel	[ˈbaʊəl]	n. 肠；内部
syndrome	[ˈsɪndrəʊm]	n. 综合征；综合症状；典型表现
colon	[ˈkəʊlən]	n. 结肠
intracellular	[ˌɪntrəˈseɪljʊlə]	adj. 细胞内的
chlamydia	[kləˈmɪdɪə]	n. 衣原体
pneumoniae	[njuːˈməʊnɪə]	n. 肺炎；急性肺炎
phylum	[ˈfaɪləm]	n. （生物分类学上的）门
platyhelminth	[plætɪˈhelmɪnθ]	n. 扁形动物（低等蠕虫，包括涡虫、血吸虫、猪肉绦虫等）
schistosoma	[ˈʃɪstəsəʊmə]	n. 血吸虫属，裂体属，裂体吸虫属
haematobium	[hiːˈmeɪtəbjəm]	n. （pl. haematobia）血内生物，住血生物
viverrini	[vəˈverɪnɪ]	n. 吸虫
sinensis	[sɪnənsɪs]	adj. 华支的
chlonorchis		支睾吸虫属
cholangiocarcinoma	[kəʊlədʒiːəʊkɑːsɪˈnəʊm]	n. 胆管癌

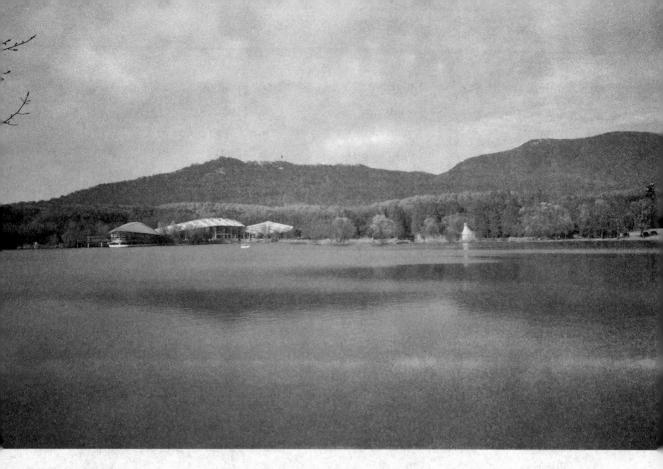

◆ Questions

1. What kind of infections are the most important causes of major types of cancer?
2. What exact percentages of infections were estimated to be associated with HCC cases attributable to HBV and to HCV according to Parkin?
3. What kind of cancer is the second most commonly diagnosed cancer in women and is the third leading cause of cancer death in women worldwide?
4. Streptococcus bovis is a normal inhabitant of the human gastrointestinal tract, so there is no connection between streptococcus bovis and the cancer, isn't there?
5. The risk of what three major viral chronic infections and bacterial (H. pylori) chronic infections are higher than that attributable to important risk factors, such as environmental pollution?

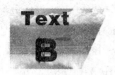

Considerations for Clinical Evaluation of Respiratory Syncytial Virus (RSV) Vaccine Candidates in RSV-naïve Infants

Jeff Roberts, MD
*Division of Vaccines and Related Product
Applications OVRR/CBER/FDA*

Good morning. I wanted to start by thanking the committee members, our presenters, the manufacturers. We are aware that preparing for a meeting like this is a lot of work. So we really appreciate you joining us today to help us think through some of the issues here as we consider moving forward with the development of these products in RSV-naive infants.

What I hope to do is, what I'm planning, is a really broad overview of the agenda, touching on each item very briefly from a high level, and I hope that's going to help frame this discussion for today. It really starts with these initial studies with the formalin-inactivated RSV vaccine candidates or FI-RSV.

These candidate vaccines were produced by growing wild-type RSV in cell culture. They are formalin-inactivated and they're adjuvant with alum. There were several studies. I'm just quoting one of them. In this particular one, infants 2 – 7 months of age were randomized either to FI-RSV or parainfluenza virus candidate vaccine, and among those subjects who were infected with RSV, 80 percent in the FI-RSV arm, compared with 5 percent of the control subjects, required hospitalization for RSV disease.

These findings were really unequivocal. There was clearly a more severe disease in the vaccinated subjects, and there were two deaths in these trials. Obviously this presented a substantial challenge for the development of RSV vaccines, and these trials were done almost exactly 50 years ago, and we still have no licensed RSV vaccine.

In the meantime, RSV epidemiology has been fairly stable, and there is a tremendous burden of disease. Just quoting some topline numbers here of global incidence per year in children less than 5. 34

million hospitalizations for lower respiratory tract infection, 3.4 million hospitalizations, and somewhere in the neighborhood of up to 200,000 deaths. In the United States, for hospitalizations, around 170,000 and an estimate of 500 deaths in the United States.

So when you think about the comparison to other infectious diseases, it's really striking that once you get outside the neonatal period and you talk about the period from 28 days to one year, RSV is second only to malaria as the leading cause of death worldwide.

There may be some other elements to this burden of disease. As an example, I've put up some data from this New England journal study with the use of palivizumab, which is a monoclonal antibody for prevention of RSV. I'll talk about it a little more in a minute.

In this study, healthy premature infants 33 to 35 weeks were randomized to placebo or palivizumab, and they had good outcomes in terms of preventing RSV, but what they also showed here is a substantial decrease in the events of recurrent wheeze over the first year of life, and a very substantial decrease in number of days with wheeze. This suggests a potential long-term impact on asthma outcomes.

Then there is, of course, the direct health care cost, and there's also sort of an unqualifiable burden parents with babies who suffer, and I think many of us are intimately familiar with that. In the face of that very substantial burden of disease, I think it's been really encouraging over recent years to see the new developments in this field of RSV vaccine development. And I think one of the really fundamental breakthroughs was the approval of RespiGam in 1996 and Synagis, or palivizumab, in 1998. This showed proof of concept that passively administered antibodies in the form of a polyclonal sera, which is RespiGam, or a monoclonal antibody product could prevent RSV.

In addition to that we've had multiple scientific and technical breakthroughs in producing improved vaccine antigens, like the pre-F protein, and then characterizing them in the vaccine technologies that are being developed to vector some of these proteins and at this point, we've got at this count at least 60 vaccines in development. So it's a pretty dizzying array of different vaccine products, and we'll talk about it a little bit more.

So it wasn't surprising, I guess, that when WHO did this landscape analysis a couple of years ago to think about where to

医学英语学术交流教程

focus their efforts, they considered criteria like the magnitude of the public health burden and the chances of success of the different products in development, and RSV really came to the top in terms of a priority for development.

I have put in this slide just to recognize that this space is really complicated and that there are—it includes the development of these candidates in many different populations, including in older adults. We have several that have advanced into late phase development. A lot of activity in maternal immunization, including one product in phase Ⅲ, but the point of this slide is to help us narrow down and focus on the specific population of RSV-naive infants and for active immunization.

What I'm recognizing here is that some of the live-attenuated vaccine products have already been studied in RSV-naive infants, and there is a substantial safety database alleviates to some degree the concern about enhanced respiratory disease. But to our knowledge, no other vaccine candidates have been studied since those initial studies in the 1960s in this specific population.

Okay, so there are many ways to divide up and think about the different vaccine technologies that are going forward, and I have this slide up because one of the things that we want the committee to think about as we move through the day is what the science can tell us potentially about these different approaches to vaccinating and potentially what elements of the scientific data could be filled in to help support the safety going forward with some of these specific technologies.

That's a really brief and broad overview, and we'll get into the details of each of these specific topics. Susan Gerber is going to tell us more detail about the latest on RSV epidemiology. Fernando Polack is going to go back and really dissect some of those initial trials with the FI-RSV and what they can tell us, and talk about the animal modeling of ERD and what each of those animal models can bring to bear.

Sarah Browne is going to give an overview of our evaluation of these data so far, and the two manufacturers here, GSK and Janssen, both have vaccine candidates that they intend to develop in RSV-naive infants. They both have a substantial package of preclinical data to support that and the both have some clinical, some early clinical data. So they've agreed to present those programs as examples for us to help think through the issues.

Okay, what I am going to do is I am going to read these questions verbatim, because I want these to be in the committee's mind over the course of the day as we hear all these presentations, and then we'll go back to them one at a time and put them up on the screen during the committee discussion.

In the meantime, I want you to think about these discussion topics. So number one is please discuss the preclinical data essential to support studies of RSV vaccines in RSV-naive infants, with regard to the potential risk of vaccine-associated ERD. Please consider the impact of vaccine type, antigen, and/or other relevant factors.

Number two is please discuss the role of clinical data from adults and RSV-experienced infants to support the evaluation of RSV vaccines in the RSV-naïve infants.

Number three is please discuss how studies in RSV-naïve infants could be designed to mitigate concerns about ERD throughout clinical development, including please consider aspects of initial study design such as eligibility criteria, age de-escalation, and duration of follow-up. Please consider relevant aspects of phase III study design.

That's all I have for now, and I think we can probably go straight into the next presentation.

(1356 words)

※ The text is extracted from Vaccines and Related Biological Products Advisory Committee May 17, 2017; Jeff Roberts, MD; Division of Vaccines and Related Product Applications OVRR/CBER/FDA

Part Ⅲ   Oral Practice

Practice 1
Clinical Inquiry—Department of Pediatrics

 Vocabulary

morbilli	[mɔːˈbɪlaɪ]	*n.* [内科]麻疹 an acute and highly contagious viral disease marked by distinct red spots followed by a rash; occurs primarily in children
rubeola	[ruˈbiːələ]	*n.* 麻疹
rubella	[ruˈbelə]	*n.* [内科]风疹 a contagious viral disease that is a milder form of measles lasting three or four days; can be damaging to a fetus(胎儿) during the first trimester 三个月
varicella	[ˌværɪˈselə]	*n.* [内科]水痘 an acute contagious disease caused by herpes(疱疹)
zoster		*n.* 带状疱疹 virus; causes a rash of vesicles on the face and body
parotitis	[ˌpærəˈtaɪtɪs]	*n.* [口腔]腮腺炎 inflammation of one or both parotid glands(腮腺)
pertussis	[pəˈtʌsɪs]	*n.* [内科]百日咳 a disease of the respiratory mucous membrane
laryngotracheitis	[ləˈrɪŋɡəʊˌtreɪkɪˈaɪtɪs]	*n.* 喉气管炎 the combination of the following two conditions: laryngitis and tracheitis
scarlatina	[ˌskɑːləˈtiːnə]	*n.* [内科]猩红热 an acute communicable disease (usually in children) characterized by fever and a red rash
tetanus	[ˈtet(ə)nəs]	*n.* [内科]破伤风;强直 1. an acute and serious infection of the central nervous system caused by bacterial infection of open wounds; spasms of the jaw and laryngeal muscles may occur during the late stages;

2. a sustained muscular contraction resulting from a rapid series of nerve impulses

poliomyelitis [ˌpəʊlɪəʊmaɪəˈlaɪtɪs] *n.* ［内科］脊髓灰质炎；［医］小儿麻痹症 an acute viral disease marked by inflammation of nerve cells of the brain stem and spinal cord

asthma [ˈæsmə] *n.* ［内科］［中医］哮喘，气喘 a lung condition that causes difficulty in breathing

inhaler [ɪnˈheɪlə] *n.* ［临床］吸入器；空气过滤器 a dispenser that produces a chemical vapor to be inhaled in order to relieve nasal congestion

 ## Using Lay Terms in Explanations

Explanations should be given in words the patients will understand，avoiding medical terms. Using lay terms—words familiar to people without medical knowledge—can help patients understand explanations. e. g. :

Medical Terms	Lay Terms
morbilli/rubeola	measles
rubella	German measles
varicella	chickenpox
infectious parotitis	mumps
pertussis	whooping cough
acute laryngotracheitis	croup
scarlatina	scarlet fever
tetanus	lockjaw
poliomyelitis	polio

Sample Dialogue

(asthma)

Doctor：Could you tell me, Mrs. Smith, when James started coughing?

Mother：Well, it started a week ago and it's particularly bad at night, he keeps the whole family up.

Doctor：Do you think he's having any problem with choking?

Mother：Well, he seems to be experiencing quite a lot of trouble getting his air in and catching his breath.

Doctor：Is it the first time that James has found it difficult to get it breath?

Mother：No, this has happened three times before.

Doctor：How frequently do you think it occurs?

Mother：Well, as I said, it happened about three times.

Doctor: Have you noticed any relationship to the time of the year? Is it more likely to happen in the spring, for instance, rather than in the winter?

Mother: No, if anything, it's slightly more likely to happen in winter.

Doctor: And have you noticed anything else that brings it on?

Mother: Yes, I have, it always seems to be associated with a cold.

Doctor: Have you noticed anything else, such as, does it start when he's running about or when he's been in contact with animals or anything like that?

Mother: No, I haven't, although I must admit he's not very athletic and he does complain sometimes when he's running about a lot. It makes him cough and particularly in cold weather.

Doctor: Has he had any treatment for this?

Mother: Yes, he has had some treatment every now and then, he has had an inhaler which has helped a little bit.

Doctor: What about the present episode? What treatment has he had for this?

Mother: Well, he's not had anything for this one because I was hoping it would just settle on its own.

Doctor: And with the present episode, how difficult has it been to get it breath? Has he been able to talk to you all right?

Mother: It's been so difficult to catch his breath that he couldn't speak clearly to me.

Doctor: Has he looked blue or pale?

Mother: No, not that I remember.

Doctor: And how long did that last?

Mother: I'd say it lasted around five minutes. It was very scary.

Doctor: Has this been difficulty that's made him lose time from school?

Mother: He hasn't been to school for three days this week.

 Practice 2

International Conference—Introducing a Conference and Making Requests to the Audience

 Useful Expressions for Introducing a Conference

1. We are here today to ...
2. Our main aim today is to ...
3. The conference will be held every year to make it an ideal platform for people to

share views and experiences.

4. The conference aims to bring together researchers, scientists, the practical challenges encountered and the solutions adopted.

5. This summit will provide opportunity for academic exchange and contribute to the development of ...

6. The goals of this conference are twofold. First, it should ... Second, it should ...

7. The history of this gathering/conference goes back to ... when it first became apparent to us that developments in the field of ... become so important that a conference seemed mandatory.

8. It is the aim of this conference to bring together mainly those who have contributed over a period of years to this subject.

9. Our purpose here is to define the present status of knowledge concerning ... in five different fields. First, ... Second, ... Third, ... Fourth, ... finally, ...

10. This conference will focus on the discussion of the various aspects of ...

11. If we are all here, let's get started/start the meeting/start.

12. I am very pleased and honored to declare ... (the conference) open.

13. Now I declare the ... conference is open! Please allow me to introduce today's speakers.

14. It is a great pleasure for me to welcome you to Session on ...

15. It gives me pleasure to welcome you to Session on ...

16. It is a privilege for me to welcome you to Session on ...

17. I am privileged to welcome you to Session on ...

 Useful Expressions for Making Requests to the Audience

1. Time for discussion, do you have any questions?

2. Any more questions or comments for Dr. A?

3. Let's turn/move on to the next problem (the subject of ...)

4. I think that'll be the last/final question before we close this session/go on to the next speaker.

5. May I have your attention please?

6. Let's take five minutes stretch.

7. At the end of each presentation, there will be 5 minutes for discussion.

8. At the end of the session we will have an open discussion on any of the papers presented.

9. Sorry, the schedule is very/rather tight. We haven't any time for discussion, so we must go on to next paper.

Useful Expressions for Audience Manners

1. No talking. Unless audience participation is requested by the performers. If something must be said, whisper it quickly. Excessively shushing a talkative neighbor can be just as disturbing.

2. Use good posture. Auditorium seating is often arranged so that the person in the seat behind can see between the two seats in front, so slumping sideways or lounging on a partner's shoulder blocks the view.

3. Remove hats. Ladies, if your hat is part of your outfit, you can keep it on as long as it doesn't block anyone's view.

4. Noises off. Turn off cell phones, beepers, audible watches, and any other sound-making gadgets before any performance.

5. Lights out. Don't forget, the screen on your mobile device can be a distraction too. No rattling of candy boxes or ice in cups, shaking popcorn containers, or slurping drinks.

6. Control coughing. Muffle coughs and sneezes with a handkerchief. Cough drops and mints may be helpful, but leave if you can't stop the attack.

7. Avoid other sounds that can disturb the people around you and the performers. Munching noisily, smacking or cracking gum, rattling the pages of programs, tapping feet or drumming fingers, humming or singing along, rummaging in purses—these are just a few of the things that can annoy those around you.

8. Smoke only in designated areas. Leave and find a place outside if you must smoke.

9. Don't take flash photos or shoot video during live performances. The point is to do nothing that will distract the performers or disturb others in the audience.

10. Dispose of trash, including chewed gum, in waste containers. Tell the next user or attendant if anything was spilled, as a courtesy to the next person who has your seat.

Practice 3

Oral English for Culture and on Social Occasions
—Traditional Chinese Art Occasion: Traditional Chinese Art

Useful Expressions for Enjoying Traditional Chinese Art		
刺绣	embroidery	剪纸　Paper Cutting
对联	(Spring Festival) Couplets	书法　Calligraphy

風水　Fengshui/Geomantic Omen

红白喜事　Weddings and Funerals

武打片　Chinese Swordplay Movie

唐三彩　Tri-color Pottery of the Tang Dynasty/The Tang Tri-colored pottery

秦腔　Crying of Qin People/Qin Opera

相声　Cross-talk/Comic Dialogue

电视小品　TV Sketch/TV Skit

文房四宝(笔墨纸砚)　The Four Treasures of the Study (Brush，Ink stick，Paper，
and Ink stone)

太极拳　Tai Chi　　　　　　　　　　针灸　Acupuncture

川剧变脸　Face-changing in Sichuan Opera

Activities and Role-play (inviting students to improvise and act it out)

Sample Sentences

There is your seat.

Would you like to lower your voice?

Would you like to make some space for the lady?

Please do not smoke in the theater.

Please pay attention to the signs in the theater.

When you excuse yourself to go to the restroom, just say "Please excuse me."

Why don't you ... ?

Do you think it is a good idea ... ?

Topics for Further Discussion

1. Do you know anything about traditional Chinese art?
2. Which kind of Chinese art do you enjoy most?
3. Who is the best tradition Chinese artist in your mind?
4. Introduce one of traditional Chinese arts.
5. Differences between Chinese and American traditional festivals.

References for Further Discussion

1. Face-changing in Sichuan Opera

We cannot talk about face changing without mentioning Sichuan Opera. Sichuan Opera is one of many local operas in China, popular in the provinces of Sichuan, Yunnan and Guizhou. Face changing is not simply changing one's facial makeup in a casual way, but is a special technique in the performance of Sichuan Opera. It refers to the changing of masks in quick succession to show different emotions and feelings of the character in the play.

It is said the origin of face changing has something to do with the resistance of wild beasts. In ancient times, when coming across a ferocious animal, people used to draw different patterns on their faces to scare the animal away and keep themselves safe. Later on, such trick was applied to the stage performance of Sichuan Opera, and the unique art of face changing has thus come into being.

Face-changing techniques generally fall into three categories, "wiping（抹脸）", "blowing（吹脸）" and "pulling（扯脸）". "Wiping" is to spread the paint over the face while performing. The paint is put on a certain part of the face in advance. "Blowing" is only employed when powder cosmetics are used. On the stage, a tiny box with powder cosmetics in it is placed before hand. A movement of prostration near the box will enable the performer to blow the powder onto his face. When one is going to use the "pulling" technique he has to draw facial masks on fine pieces of silk cloth, cut them into the right size, tie a thin thread to each mask and stick them onto his face before the performance. The threads are fastened to somewhere hidden in his costumes. Many performers prefer to tie them onto their waistbands. When performing, the artist would pull the mask off one after another under the cover of various dancing movements.

In practice, the first method of the three is most employed because it is the simplest, while "blowing" is relatively more complicated since one has to close his eyes and shut up his mouth when blowing in case the powder would fly into his eyes and mouth so the performance would not be continued. However, "pulling" is the most troublesome among the three skills. The dancing movements have to be natural and the action of pulling should be invisible to the audience. If the audience see through the trick of face changing, they would probably get dissatisfied and pull a face too!

2. Culture differences make the festivals diversified. The different festivals make the world more colorful. Doing research in festivals you can find some interesting and valuable evidence to prove the uniqueness of the cultures.

The first and foremost, the Chinese festivals emphasize the value of individual and small family. In China, the festivals are the time to meet family members and share family stories. The most typical Chinese festivals are the Spring Festival, the Lantern Festival, the Dragon Boat Festival, Mid-Autumn Festival, and the Double Ninth Festival. All of them bear the same features which are the union of the family members and the memory of the ancestors. The celebration happens in private place, especially family house which is illegal to intrude. However, Western festivals pay more attention on public values and civil attitudes. No matter Las Fallas (Mar. 19th), April Fool's Day, Oktoberfest (Oct. 10), or Halloween are the festivals for all the people. During these festivals, people gather together in the open square or run through the streets to watch fireworks, to eat, and drink beers. They are totally different from Chinese counterpart.

The second distinguished difference is that they have different worships. The Chinese festivals are activities of performing superstition, taboo, and sacrifice. In the primary age, people cannot understand many natural phenomena. They are scared by the nature, so they become superstitious. They believed fireworks can frighten away beasts and created Spring Festival. There are many taboos during Spring Festival such as forbid spraying water and sweeping floor. Qing Ming Festival (Apr. 4 or 5), and Hungry Ghost Festival (lunar Jul. 15), are the festivals to perform sacrifice. The festivals are also called for "ghost festivals" for it is a custom to sacrifice domestic animals to revere ancestors. However, Christianity is pervasive almost in every aspect in western society. There are many festivals related to this religion. Epiphany (Jan. 6) shows the scholars and rulers understand God's purpose in allowing Jesus to be born on the earth. Good Friday (the Friday before Easter) is the anniversary of crucifixion of Jesus Christ. Easter (the first full moon after Mar. 21) celebrates the Christ's resurrection. Christmas Day, the 25th of December, is the biggest festival celebrated in the Christian countries of the world which symbolizes the birthday of Jesus Christ. These festivals almost cover all the great deeds of Jesus Christ which also reflect the powerful worship of Christianity.

When it comes to how to celebrate festivals, there are still some differences. The Chinese festivals pay more attention on eating and drinking. It goes so beyond that every festival has its unique food to eat, such as to eat dumplings in the Spring Festival, to eat *yuanxiao* in the Lantern Festival, and to eat mooncakes in the Mid-Autumn festival. However, the Western festivals have fun passionately. Just like the Roman philosopher Seneca said human beings cannot live without festivals, because only carnivals can help people run away from the norms and rules which fetter people to enjoy natural instincts. That is why Westerners all enjoy carnivals. During Las Fallas (Mar. 19th) people gather together to watch fireworks and drink beer to show their passion for public affairs. On April Fool's Day, you can play tricks on those people who are older or more influential than you. Either Oktoberfest, or Halloween is the festival for all the people.

Unit 6

Key Points

....

Learning Targets

- To *imitate* the speech style of the modelling speech
- To produce a *synopsis* of a passage
- To learn about the academic terms of gynecology and obstetrics in clinical diagnostic conversation

Learning Focus

- How to announce a break and the closing remarks at an international academic conference

Cultural Points

- Chinese wine culture and dining etiquette

✓音、视频资源
✓参考译文
✓参考答案
✓学术探讨

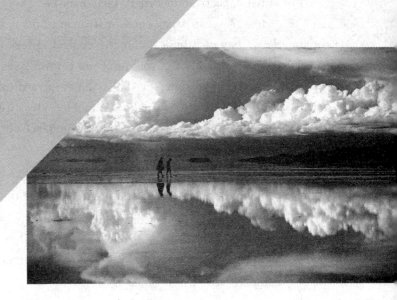

Part I　Listening Comprehension

Video 1

Beyond Inclusion—Women and Clinical Trials

Exercise I　Take notes while watching the video, and then answer the following questions.

1. What is the gender difference in the occurrence of autism between boys and girls?
2. What is the gender difference in the occurrence of asthma between boys and girls?
3. Why does the speaker cite the example of a 75-year-old woman for a study of stroke?
4. What does the speaker imply by mentioning gender difference in stroke in the latter part of her speech?

Exercise II　Take notes while watching the video, and then complete the following sentences.

For autism spectrum disorder, girls may be ___5___ from clinical trials because they're not ___6___ or ___7___. In fact, some instruments do not perform well in ___8___ girls with autism. So we have to think about the clinical criteria, what tools we use for ___9___ and tailor them appropriately to avoid omitting certain populations at risk.

As for the implications in the asthma, stratification by sex should be considered during design and analysis. Analysis should ___10___ interactions specifically between age and sex gender. And trials may ___11___ emphasis on recruitment of ages around those switch points.

Exercise III　Watch the video and decide whether the following statements are true (T) or false (F) in terms of gender difference in stroke in clinical trials.

12. Premenopausal women have more strokes than men of the same age.
13. Women have longer life expectancy and higher incidence of strokes overall compared to men at older ages.
14. Brain hemorrhage is more common in women than in men.

15. The quality of life after stroke is better in women than in men.

16. Dangers in antiplatelet therapy are definitely higher in women than in men.

Video 2 ▐▐▐▐

The Problem with Race-Based Medicine

Exercise I Fill in the blanks with the missing words or expressions.

Sociologists like me have long explained that race is a social __1__. When we identify people as black, white, Asian, Native American, Latina, we're referring to __2__ with made-up demarcations that have changed over time and vary around the world. As a legal scholar, I've also studied how lawmakers, not biologists, have invented the legal definitions of races. And it's not just the view of social scientists. Doctors are supposed to practice __3__, and they're increasingly called to join the genomic revolution. But their habit of treating patients by race lags far behind.

Take the estimate of __4__ rate, or GFR. Doctors routinely interpret GFR, this important indicator of kidney function, by race. As you can see in this lab test, the exact same creatinine level, the concentration in the blood of the patient, automatically produces a different GFR estimate depending on whether or not the patient is African-American. Why?

I've been told it's based on an assumption that African-Americans have more muscle mass than people of other races. But what sense does it make for a doctor to __5__ assume I have more muscle mass than that female bodybuilder? Wouldn't it be far more accurate and evidence-based to determine the muscle mass of individual patients just by looking at them?

Well, doctors tell me they're using race as a __6__. It's a crude but convenient proxy for more important factors, like muscle mass, __7__, genetic traits they just don't have time to look for. But race is a bad proxy. In many cases, race adds no relevant information at all. It's just a distraction. But race also tends to __8__ the clinical measures. It blinds doctors to patients' symptoms, family illnesses, their history, their own illnesses they might have—all more evidence-based than the patients' race. Race can't __9__ these important clinical measures without sacrificing patients' well-being.

Doctors also tell me race is just one of many factors they take into account, but there are numerous medical tests, like the GFR, that use race __10__ to treat black, white, Asian patients differently just because of their race.

Exercise Ⅱ   Watch the video and decide whether the following statements are true (T) or false (F).

11. Race influences all the medical practice，according to the speaker.

12. Race is actually more important than clinical measures.

13. Doctors often treat patients differently because of their races.

14. Race-based medicine is not simply a medical problem.

Listing 1

Mechanism of Painkillers

Exercise Ⅰ   Crossword the following words based on what you've heard. You may refer to the hints in the Across-Down region below if necessary.

install	stimulus	block	rinse	sensation
spine	dimension	nociceptor	fire	threshold

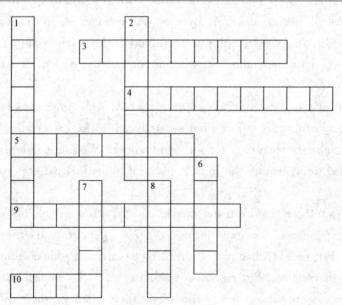

ACROSS

3   a feeling that you get when something affects your body and the ability to feel through your sense of touch

DOWN

1   an aspect of or a category of things distinguished by some common characteristic or quality

4 an amount, level, or limit on a scale and when it is reached, something else happens or changes

5 something that produces a reaction or encourages activity in a human, an animal or a plant

9 a type of receptor at the end of a sensory neuron's axon that responds to damaging or potentially damaging stimuli by sending pain signals to the spinal cord

10 to function or work, or to make something such as a device, a chemical process or a biological unit start working

2 to fit something or put it at a specific place so that it is ready to be used for some special purpose

6 to prevent something from happening, developing, producing or making progress

7 to wash something with clean water only, not using soap or to remove dirt or sand, etc. from something by washing it with clean water

8 any of the sharp pointed parts like needles on some plants and animals

Exercise Ⅱ Fill in the blanks with the original words and phrases or with expressions which have the same or the closest meaning.

11. A person could get hurt, or even hurt himself but never knows it if he can't feel pain, because pain is our body's _____ system.

12. Detectors of nociceptors are specialized nerve cells which can stretch from your _____, to your _____, your _____, your _____, your _____, and some of your internal organs.

13. The _____ you push against the needle, the _____ you get to the nociceptors threshold.

14. Once cells are damaged, they and other nearby cells start producing these _____ chemicals like crazy, lowering the nociceptors' _____ to the point where gentle touch can cause pain.

15. _____, acting like a spine from a porcupine, enters the active sites of COX – 1 and COX – 2 and then breaks off, leaving half of itself in there, totally _____ that channel and making it impossible for the arachidonic acid to fit.

Listening 2

Side-effect of Drugs on Females

Exercise I   Choose correct answers to the following questions.

1. As an emergency medicine doctor, what problem did the speaker found in practice?
   A. Too many patients need emergency medicine service.
   B. She found it difficult to try her best to save people's life.
   C. She orders tests and prescribes medications without thinking about patient's gender.
   D. There is a shortage of medical service and medication.

2. How many drugs were withdrawn from the market because of the side effects on women?
   A. 80%   B. 90%   C. 20%   D. 50%

3. According to the speech, if women take the same dose of Ambien as men do, what will happen?
   A. They will vomit in the morning.
   B. They will suffer severe headache the next day.
   C. They will still feel sleepy the next morning.
   D. They will feel like committing suicide the next morning.

4. According to the speaker, one of the things that World War II changed was _____.
   A. the great deduction of the population around the world
   B. more people voluntarily attending the medical research
   C. the war destroying most of the medical service in the world
   D. people not having to fear being victims of medical research

5. Why did scientists only use men and male animals as subjects of medical researches?
   A. Because males are stronger than females.
   B. Because there were more males than females after World War II.
   C. Because men tend to be more interested in medical research than women.
   D. Because scientists feared that the medical studies might do harm to women's fetus.

Exercise II   Listen to the material and decide whether the following statements are true (T) or false (F).

6. Most of the medical discoveries in the past century were on the basis of studies on

医学英语学术交流教程

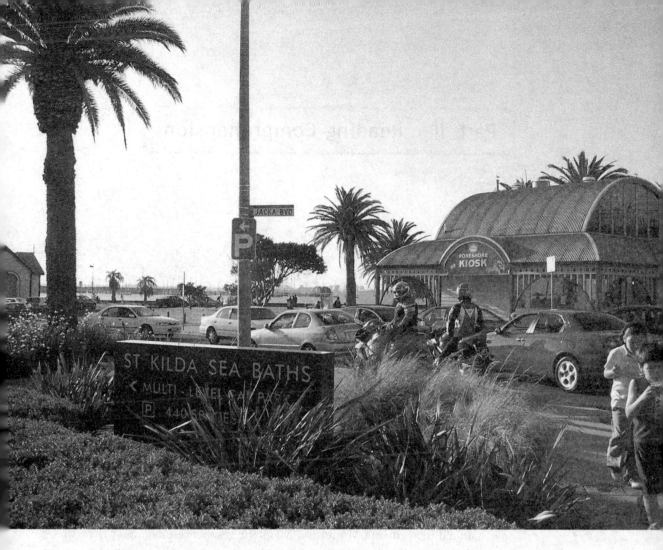

the whole population.

7. Some medication we prescribed to women may have side effects on them.

8. A drug must be tested on animals before it is prescribed to human patients.

9. According to the speech, Ambien is not suitable for women because women have fewer sleeping disorders.

10. Usually, women metabolize the drug at a faster rate than men.

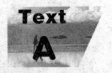

Case No. 154：32-year-old Computer Software Engineer with Nodular Mass in the Liver （1）

Elisabeth Fabian
Presentation of Case

Dr. W. Spindelboeck:

Due to episodic epigastric pain this 32-year-old woman had undergone computed tomography （CT） 20 months previously. Contrast enhanced CT showed a hypodense lesion between liver segments Ⅳ and Ⅷ with a diameter of 4 cm and inhomogenous early enhancement suggesting hemangioma. Eight more lesions （diameter up to 1 cm） that were only visible in the early arterial phase were found in segments Ⅵ and Ⅲ. Magnetic resonance imaging （MRI） 13 and 8 months before admission showed slight progression （from a diameter of 4. 0 to 4. 6 cm） of the lesion in segment Ⅳ. At that time, the lesion appeared to be lobulated with a central hyper intense scar and arterial enhancement, primarily compatible with "atypical" focal nodular hyperplasia （FNH）. Except for occasional abdominal pain and a 10-year history of histamine intolerance, the patient was free of symptoms. She had taken thyroid replacement therapy （Euthyrox * 100 μg per day） for years. She had no previous surgery, never received a blood transfusion, and was not vaccinated against hepatitis A or B. She neither smoked nor drank and her family history was unremarkable. The patient is a single parent of a healthy 10-year-old boy. Physical examination was unremarkable. She weighed 56 kg and her height was 174 cm. Except for lactate dehydrogenase （LDH: 296 U/l, normal 120—240 U/l） routine laboratory tests were negative. A panel of antibodies to detect autoimmune and collagen vascular diseases was negative; thyroid stimulating hormone （TSH） was 1. 3 μU/ml （normal 0. 1—4. 0 μU/

l). During a follow-up exam in the outpatient liver clinic, she showed a facial flush that lasted for 2 min, although the situation was not psychologically upsetting. She said facial flushes are part of her histamine intolerance. A diagnostic test was performed, and she was admitted to the hospital for further management.

Differential Diagnosis
Dr. B. Haas:

The patient under discussion is a 32-year old woman with nodules in the liver. Except for occasional abdominal pain and histamine intolerance, she is asymptomatic. Twenty months earlier, CT of the liver showed what was first thought to be a hemangioma and later interpreted as an "atypical" FNH. Further MRIs revealed progression of the lesion (from a diameter of 4.0 to 4.6 cm) and identified eight additional lesions (diameter up to 1 cm) in the liver. Facial flushes were thought by the patient to be due to histamine intolerance diagnosed 10 years before. Physical examination did not show any abnormality and, except for LDH, routine laboratory tests were within normal limits. As the patient is a native of Austria, hepatocellular carcinoma (HCC) in a noncirrhotic liver due to chronic hepatitis B is unlikely. Since hepatitis serology is routinely tested during pregnancy in this country, an infection would have been revealed much earlier when the patient had been pregnant. It is unclear whether the patient had consumed foods such as wild berries or raw vegetables and so might have been infected with echinococcus. However, the MRI lesions are not typical for echinococcal cysts. An infection with Bartonella henselae due to contact with cats and a resulting bacillary peliosis hepatis could be considered, but this disease predominantly occurs in immunosuppressed patients, is associated with fever, and runs a much shorter course. As to the episodic abdominal pain, a regular recurrence of symptoms could parallel the menstrual cycle, but endometriosis would not really explain the liver lesions. Since the panel of antibodies for autoimmune and collagen vascular diseases was negative, an autoimmune disease can also be ruled out. The patient said she was histamine intolerant, but unfortunately no further information was available as to how this diagnosis was established 10 years earlier. FNH could still be considered as a possible diagnosis, but it would not have required prompt admission to the hospital. The assumed diagnosis of a liver hemangioma based on the CT scan, which showed a hypodense lesion with inhomogenous early arterial contrast enhancement, appears unlikely since the lesion had progressed in size.

For my differential diagnosis, I have to address the facial flush presumed to be due to histamine intolerance. Flush symptoms can be caused by enhanced release of vasoactive substances such as serotonin and bradykinin, mostly due to a gastroenteropancreatic neuroendocrine tumor (GEP-NET). Frequently, flush symptoms in GEP-NETs occur in the setting of liver metastases. This is because most of the bioactive substances that are released by a GEP-NET may be metabolized by the liver on first pass from the splanchnic area and, more importantly, liver metastases provide for more tissue for production and release of bioactive substances into the circulation. Laboratory tests showed elevated serum LDH, with an increased ratio of LDH/AST, a possible marker for the presence of liver metastases. An important diagnostic test that could suggest a GEP-NET is the analysis of serum chromogranin A. Chromogranin A is a protein found in the secretory granules of neuroendocrine cells, and its concentration correlates with tumor mass. Further diagnostic steps include analysis of 5-hydroxyindol acetic acid (5-HIAA) in a 24-h urine sample. Endoscopic investigation including capsule endoscopy of the small bowel, abdominal sonography, and contrast-enhanced CT, PET, and radionuclear imaging such as 99m technetium octreotid scintigraphy and 68gallium-DOTATATE (= DOTADOC) PET-CT are parts of the further workup.

(862 words)

※ The text is extracted from *Clinical-Pathological Conference Series from the Medical University of Graz*.

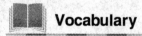

Vocabulary

epigastric	[epɪˈɡæstrɪk]	*adj.* 腹上部的
inhomogenous	[ˈɪnhəmədʒɪnəs]	*adj.* 不均一的；多相的；异成分的
hemangioma	[hɪːˌmændʒiːˈəʊmə]	*n.* 血管瘤
lobulate	[ˈlɒbjʊleɪt]	*adj.* 由小叶片组成的，分成小裂片的
histamine	[ˈhɪstəmiːn]	*n.* 组胺
dehydrogenase	[diːˈhaɪdrədʒəneɪs]	*n.* 脱氢酶
asymptomatic	[ˌeɪsɪmptəˈmætɪk]	*adj.* 无临床症状的

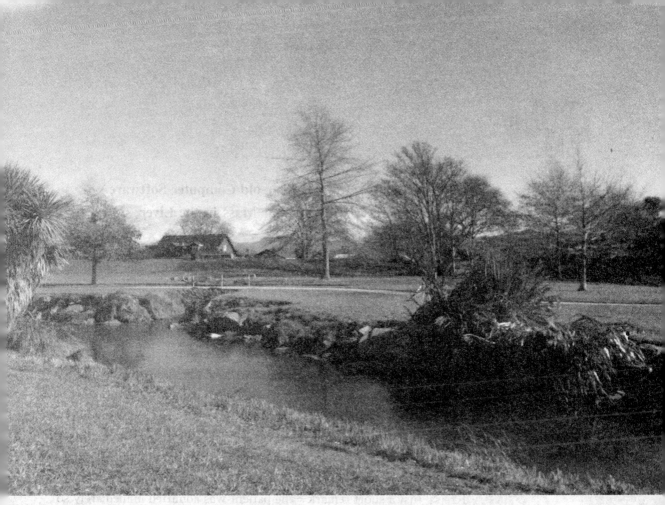

cirrhotic	[sɪˈrɒtɪk]	*adj.* 肝脏硬化症的
echinococcus	[ˌɪkaɪnəˈkɒkəs]	*n.* 棘球绦虫
peliosis	[ˌpiːlɪˈəʊsɪs]	*n.* 紫癜
endometriosis	[ˌendəʊˌmiːtrɪˈəʊsɪs]	*n.* 子宫内膜异位
diamine oxidase	[daɪˈæmiːn ˈɒksɪdeɪs]	*n.* 二胺氧化酶
splanchnic	[ˈsplæŋknɪk]	*adj.* 内脏的
chromogranin	[krəʊməʊɡˈrænɪn]	*n.* 嗜铬粒蛋白
scintigraphy	[sɪnˈtɪɡrəfɪ]	*n.* 闪烁扫描法

◆ Questions

1. What is wrong with the 32-year-old patient?
2. What symptoms does the patient have?
3. What did the patient's physical examination show?
4. Why is the patient unlikely to have the chronic hepatitis B induced HCC?
5. What did the patient say about her facial flushes?
6. What did Dr. B. Haas think about the facial flush?
7. What steps did Dr. B. Haas suggest should be included in further diagnosis?

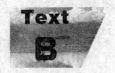

Text B

Case No. 154: 32-year-old Computer Software Engineer with Nodular Mass in the Liver (2)

Elisabeth Fabian
Discussion of Diagnosis

Dr. W. Spindelboeck:

This patient does indeed have a gut neuroendocrine tumor (NET). Further history revealed that flush symptoms as noticed in the outpatient liver clinic occur 10 to 50 times per day. The patient complained of bloating but denied diarrhea. The following laboratory results were obtained:

Serum chromogranin A 1061 ng/ml (normal 0—99 ng/ml), serum serotonin 2063 ng/ml (normal 80—450 ng/ml), and urinary 5-HIAA 118 mg/24h (normal 6—10 mg/24h). For further staging, MRI of the small intestine and the liver was performed. Dr. G. J. Krejs: Just a short remark—the patient was admitted immediately so that somatostatin analog therapy could begin without delay.

Some epidemiological facts: Although previously regarded as rare, GEP-NETs represent the second most common digestive malignancy after adenocarcinomas. Based on data of the Surveillance, Epidemiology and End Results (SEER) program of the National Cancer Institute including 29,664 patients, the incidence is estimated to be 3.65/100,000 persons per year. In Austria, Dr. Niederle found a similar incidence. The incidence of GEP-NET has increased in recent decades; the expanding use of sophisticated imaging studies is believed to play a role in this development, but there seems to be a true increase. GEP-NETs mostly occur in the small intestine (31 %), followed by rectum (26 %), colon (18 %), pancreas (12 %), and appendix (6 %). The presence of liver metastases depends on the site of the primary tumor, tumor extent (T-stage), histological differentiation, and proliferative activity (grading; G1—G3). Pancreas, right hemicolon, and small intestine are the most frequent primary tumor sites presenting with distant metastases upon initial diagnosis. Some data show that 80%—90 % of patients with small intestinal neuroendocrine neoplasia also have liver metastases. In patients with "carcinoid syndrome", distant metastases are regularly observed, and they are found more frequently in patients with poorly differentiated endocrine carcinoma (NEC G3) than in those with well-differentiated NET G1—G2. Metastases in NET patients can only be assessed with sensitive imaging techniques. In addition to MRI, radio nuclear imaging was also performed in the discussed patient, and Dr. Lipp will show the results.

Dr. R. Lipp:

NET cells express somatostatin receptors (SSR) which are the target for radionuclear tracers during somatostatin-receptor scintigraphy (SSRS). For SSRS, a gamma emitter (single-photon emission CT, SPECT) such as 111In-DTPA-octreotide (OctreoScan™) and 99mTctektrotyde, or a positron emitter (positron emission tomography, PET) such as 68Ga-octreotide, 68Ga-DOTATOC, and 64Cu-DOTA-TATE is used. 18Fluro-DOPA PET/CT is another radionuclear method to assess the metabolic activity of GEP-NET cells independent of the SSR status. In NET cells the activity of DOPA-decarboxylase that decarboxylates the amin precursor DOPA to a biogenic amin is increased. Depending on the degree of differentiation, GEP-NET cells take up and metabolize 18fluro-DOPA differently. In one third of GEP-NET patients this investigation provides pivotal and therapeutically important information that cannot be obtained by other morphologic and functional imaging methods.

Dr. M. Fuchsjäger:

Radiologic imaging currently lacks specificity for GEP-NETs, which are often mistaken for more common lesions. Due to their highly variable appearance, NET liver metastases may first be taken for benign lesions such as adenoma or hemangioma or confused with another hepatic malignancy such as HCC or cholangiocarcinoma. Since these imaging findings may overlap with other liver neoplasms, diagnosis of liver metastases from NETs still rests primarily on pathological analysis and immunochemistry of biopsy and/or surgical specimens. Liver metastases seen on CT images most frequently are less attenuated than surrounding liver parenchyma on pre-contrast images but strongly enhance post-contrast, mimicking hemangioma. Metastases of NETs may be difficult to identify and delineate on CT as they may be isodense with the liver on portal venous phase

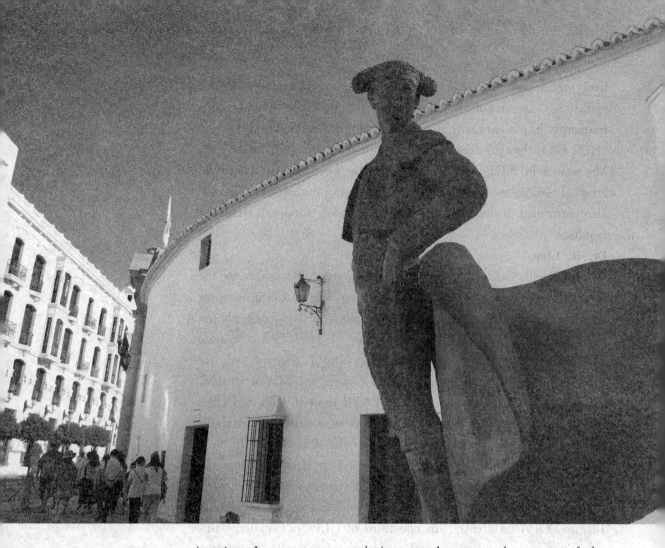

imaging. In some cases, a lesion may be seen only on one of the three phases (pre-contrast, arterial phase, and portal venous phase). MRI has a higher sensitivity for identifying the primary tumor. Tumors usually have low signal intensity on T1-weighted sequences (75%) and high signal intensity on T2-weighted sequences (94%), being hypervascular on arterial post-gadolinium images; 15% of liver metastases were only seen on the immediate post-gadolinium images. The tumors are most conspicuous on fat-suppressed T1-weighted images. Both CT and MRI can be used to stage nodal and distant metastatic disease as part of preoperative planning.

Final Diagnosis

Three neuroendocrine tumors of the ileum (G1, "carcinoids") with metastases to the mesenteric lymph nodes and the liver.

(730 words)

※ The text is extracted from *Clinical-Pathological Conference Series from the Medical University of Graz*.

Practice 1
Clinical Inquiry—Department of Gynecology and Obstetrics

 Vocabulary

belly	['belɪ]	*n.* 肚子 the underpart of the body of certain vertebrates
bend the knees		屈膝
conscious	['kɒnʃəs]	*adj.* 神志清楚的 able to use senses and mental powers to understand what is happening
mmHg		毫米汞柱(液压单位)(*abbr.*) millimeter(s) of mercury
bilateral	[ˌbaɪ'lætərəl]	*adj.* (身体部位)两侧的，对称的，(大脑)两半球的 involving both of two parts or sides of the body or brain
abdomen	['æbdəmən]	*n.* 腹部 the part of the body below the chest that contains the stomach, bowels, etc.
palpation	[pæl'peɪʃən]	*n.* 触诊，扪诊 a method of examination in which the examiner feels the size or shape or firmness or location of body parts
tenderness	['tendənɪs]	*n.* 压痛 a pain that is felt, as when the area is touched
rebound tenderness		反跳痛
masses	['mæsɪz]	*n.* 包块 an amount of something, especially a large amount which has no definite shape
bowel sound		肠鸣音
ectopic pregnancy		异位妊娠 development of a fertilized egg elsewhere than in the uterus (as in a fallopian tube or the peritoneal cavity)
shifting dullness		移动性浊音

hemorrhage	[ˈhemərɪdʒ]	*n.* 出血 a medical condition in which there is severe loss of blood from inside a person's body
threshold volume		阈值
ascites	[æˈsaɪts]	*n.* 腹水 accumulation of serous fluid in peritoneal cavity
internal bleeding		腹腔内出血
free fluid		游离液体
percussion	[pəˈkʌʃn]	*n.* 叩诊 tapping a part of the body for diagnostic purposes
negative	[ˈnegətɪv]	*adj.* (*abbr.* Neg.) 结果为阴性的（或否定的）not showing any evidence of a particular substance or medical condition
period	[ˈpɪəriəd]	*n.* 月经 the flow of blood each month from the body of a woman who is not pregnant
missed period		停经
vaginal	[vəˈdʒaɪnl]	*adj.* 阴道的 relating to or involving vagina
uterus	[ˈjuːtərəs]	*n.* 子宫 womb of a woman or female mammal
cervical lifting pain		宫颈举痛
TVS		经阴道B超(*abbr.*) a transvaginal ultrasound
lump	[lʌmp]	*n.* 包块 something hard of solid, usually without a particular shape
cul-de-sac		*n.* [医]后穹窿
culdocentesis	[kʌldəsenˈtiːsɪs]	*n.* 后穹窿穿刺术 an important and efficient method in the differential diagnosis of gynecologic acute abdomen
PID		盆腔炎(*abbr.*) pelvic inflammatory disease
intraperitoneal hemorrhage		腹腔内出血
pelvic hemorrhage		盆腔出血
rupture	[ˈrʌptʃə(r)]	*v.* 破裂 burst or break apart something inside the body
laparoscopy	[ˌlæpəˈrɒskəpi]	*n.* 腹腔镜术 an operation performed with a laparoscope that makes a small incision to examine the abdominal cavity（especially the ovaries and fallopian tubes）
transabdominal operation		经腹手术
methotrexate (MTX) injection		氨甲喋呤注射
mifepristone administration		米非司酮给药
fallopian tube		输卵管 also tuba uterina, the two tubes in a

woman's body along which eggs pass from her ovaries to her womb

 ## Using Lay Terms in Explanations

Explanations should be given in words the patients can understand. Medical Terms must be avoided on purpose. Using lay terms—words familiar to people without medical knowledge—can help patients understand explanations. e. g. :

Medical Terms	Lay Terms
1. palpation	tactual exploration
2. hemorrhage	bleeding
3. ascites	water belly
4. percussion	tapping
5. urine	liquid waste
6. menstruation	period
7. uterus	womb

Sample Dialogue

(In the ward)

Doctor: Hello, Mrs. White. How are you feeling today?

Patient: Hi, doctor Pan. I'm still feeling that pain in my belly.

Doctor: Could I give you an examination?

Patient: Sure. Thanks.

Doctor: Well, would you please bend your knees? I'm going to examine you.

Patient: OK.

Doctor: The patient is conscious and breathes smoothly at a rate of 16 breaths per minute. Her pulse rate is 90 beats per minute and the BP is 110/70 mmHg. There's nothing special with the bilateral lungs or the heart. The abdomen feels soft. Now Mrs. White, I'm going to do the palpation. Please let me know where you feel the pain.

Patient: Here, the left.

Doctor: Then what about the pain if my hand left it?

Patient: Oh, it became even more.

Doctor: Well, there's tenderness and rebound tenderness in the lower left belly. No masses have been touched. The bowel sounds haven't been heard. You know, it's the pain that made you come here, and you're diagnosed as ectopic pregnancy, we should think of the possibility of hemorrhage that can be detected through shift dullness if it reaches the threshold volume. We can't rule out ascites or internal bleeding if the shift dullness is negative. But we have to check if we suspect there's free fluid in the abdomen. Now I'll examine the shift dullness. Mrs. White, could you lie on the left side. (*Percussion*) Now the other side, please. (*Percussion*) Shift dullness is negative in this patient. We should also pay attention to the bladder at the same time. You know, sometimes the dullness you've got actually comes from the urine in it. All right. Thank you for your cooperation, Mrs. White. Things do not seem very serious, so take it easy and have a rest. See you.

Patient: Bye, doctor.

(In the doctor's office)

Chief physician: Dr. Black, could you tell me why did you make the diagnosis of ectopic pregnancy?

Intern A: Firstly, missed period, abdominal pain and vaginal bleeding are three typical syndromes of ectopic pregnancy and the patient had two of them. Secondly, vaginal examination showed normal size uterus and cervical lifting pain as well as severe tenderness on the left side. What's more, the urine pregnancy test was positive, but TVS showed an empty uterus and a lump in the left side with free fluid in the cul-de-sac. Last but the most important is the positive result of culdocentesis. So I think the evidence of ectopic pregnancy is enough.

Chief physician: Absolutely correct. Also the patient had a PID history one year ago which is the risk factor of this onset. Dr. Patrick, do you think this patient had an intraperitoneal hemorrhage?

Intern B: I think so. She had abdominal pain, tenderness, rebound tenderness, cervical lifting pain, and fluid in the cul-de-sac showed by TVS. All suggest pelvic hemorrhage.

Chief physician: Good. At present the methods of treatment include operation and medicine. If the tube is ruptured and there is pelvis hemorrhage, the patient needs emergency operation. We can select the laparoscopy or transabdominal operation. Whether to preserve the tube or not depends on the patient's requirement of productive ability. If the tube remains intact and the lump is small, and the β-HCG level is relatively low, we can choose methotrexate (MTX) injection or mifepristone administration, but meanwhile we must monitor the β-HCG level.

Intern A: I see, Professor, and then the patient is going to be operated, isn't she?

Chief physician: I think so. Dr. Patrick, have you ordered the operation?

Resident: Yes. We have made an appointment of a laparoscopy at 11:00. If the tube remains unruptured, we will choose the method of preserving the fallopian

医学英语学术交流教程

tube.

Chief physician: Very good. That's all for this case. Now let's prepare for the operation.

Resident: Thank you, Professor. See you in the operating room.

Practice 2

International Conference
—Announcing a Break and Closing Ceremony

Useful Expressions for Announcing a Coffee Break

1. We're now going to have a 15-minute break.
2. Let's take a 20-minute coffee break.
3. The session will now recess for a coffee break.
4. I'd like to declare a 15-minute recess.

Useful Expressions for Adjourning the Meeting

1. We have come to the end of our session.
2. We'll now close the session. Thank you.
3. I declare the session closed.

Useful Expressions for Ending a Speech

Signaling the Beginning of the End Part:

Well, that brings me to the end of my presentation. The last slide is brief summary of what I have talked about.

Before I stop/finish, let me just say …

To close my speech, I'll show you the last slide.

Summarizing

Let me just run over the key points again.

I'll briefly summarize the main issues.

To sum up, …

Briefly, …

In summary, definite evidence has been obtained indicating the existence of a

147

radioactive substance in the sample.

To summarize, I have talked about three aspects of the cancer problem: ...

Finally, as a summary statement, I would like to sum up the major points I have made.

Concluding

As you can see, there are some very good reasons ...

To sum up, my conclusion is that the present program is the best one.

Let me conclude my talk with the following comments.

Allow me to conclude by listing out all the factors influencing the efficacy.

In conclusion, I would like to point out the following aspects.

I'd like to leave you with the following conclusion.

Quoting

Let me close by quoting Dr. Einstein, the famous physicist, who said that, ...

I would like to come to a close by quoting what Sir Issac Newton once said, ...

Closing

That's all. Thank you, Mr. Chairman. Thank you all.

That's the end of my presentation.

So much for my speech. Thank you.

Thank you for your attention.

Thank you for your listening.

Well, I think this might be a good place for me to wind up my speech. Thank you, everyone.

The themes I have dealt with can be summarized as follows. First,... Second,... Last but not least, ... That's all for my talk. Please don't hesitate to put forward your suggestions and advice, if you have any. Thank you.

As time is limited, I can just give you the outline of what we have been studying. For any questions to be raised, I'm quite willing to discuss them with you at any time. Thank you.

That's all for my speech. If there're any points that I didn't make clearly, please point them out and I would like to give further explanations.

 Useful Expressions for Closing Ceremony

Host

In closing the International Symposium of ... let me first of all express sincere appreciation to ... for their generous support, and to all the participants for their active cooperation, without which it would have been impossible to organize the symposium and to bring it to a successful conclusion.

Speaker

On behalf of all those who have come to this Congress from abroad, I would like to thank our Italian hosts for their immense labors in organizing what has been an unsurpassed and indeed unique occasion. Our meetings were held in this artistic and historic city—this is something we shall remember to the end of our lives. Our admiration and gratitude to Professor ... and his colleagues are boundless, and we are left with a deep affection for Italy and its people.

Announcing time and address of the next meeting

I am honored to have the privilege of announcing that the next ... will be held in China in July, 2020. We should of course welcome as many scientists as possible who may be interested in it. We look forward to seeing you in Beijing. We are sure you will not be disappointed.

Closing speech

On behalf of all the members of our Organizing Committee, I wish to express our sincere gratitude/thanks to all of you who have so actively participated in this Congress to make it such a success. I now extend best wishes to all of you as you return home and to work. I look forward to seeing you again at our next Congress three years hence in Tokyo. I now declare the Congress officially closed.

Activities and Role-play (inviting students to improvise and act it out)

Practice 3 ||||

Oral English for Culture and on Social Occasions
—Wine Culture and Dining Etiquette

Useful Expressions for Wine Culture	
yellow liquor	黄酒 Brewed directly from grains; Clear, brown, or reddish-brown in color; Less than 20% alcohol
rice liquor	米酒 Generic name for fermented rice wine; Muddy in color; About 12—19.5 alcohol
Huadiao liquor	花雕酒 Brewed from glutinous rice and wheat; Clear in color; About 16% alcohol

cooking wine	料酒 Lower grade of yellow liquor; Widely used in cuisine cooking; Less that 20% alcohol
white liquor/white alcohol	白酒 A type of Chinese alcoholic beverage; Distilled from grains such as glutinous rice, sorghum, wheat, barely, millet, etc.; Over 40% alcohol
beer	啤酒 Brewed from starches (mainly cereals); Light yellow in color; About 2.5—7.5% alcohol
finger guessing	猜拳
heavy drinker	酒鬼
force others to drink	劝酒
quit drinking	戒酒

Sample Sentences

1. What would you like to drink?
2. May I fill your glass again?
3. Drink more.
4. Cheers! To your health.
5. Here's to our friendship. Cheers!
6. To the success of your trip!
7. I'm unable to drink, but thank you.
8. Bottoms up.
9. Let's make a toast.
10. I don't want to drink anything with alcohol.
11. My wife drives me to drink.
12. Make it two.
13. Make that a double, please.
14. Let's go bar-hopping.
15. Let's drink till me drop.
16. I am still sober.
17. I am stone/cold sober.
18. I am drunk.

Useful Expressions for Dining Etiquette

etiquette 礼仪	chopstick 筷子
toasting 举杯祝酒	guest 客人
generosity 慷慨	hospitality 好客

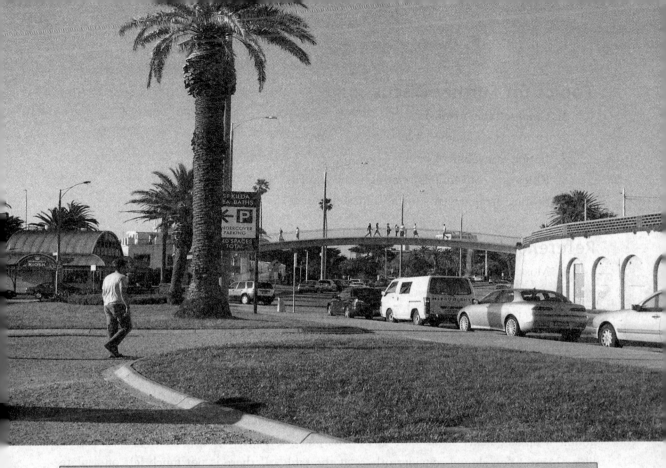

Sample Sentences

1. Help yourself.
2. Have some more.
3. Have more.
4. Have a little more.
5. Eat more.
6. Would you like a little bite more?
7. Please pass the salt.
8. If you don't like fish, just set it aside.
9. I'd like to have another helping, thanks.
10. Ah, here come the egg rolls.
11. Try some of the cold dishes.
12. Another course is coming up.
13. Just help yourself to whatever you'd like.
14. Since you don't help yourself, I'll help you with some fish balls.
15. It tastes best when taken piping hot.
16. May I help you get some pieces of sweet sour fish?
17. What a delicious meal! Thank you very much.
18. Thank you. But I really can't eat another bite.

Topics for Further Discussion

1. Chinese table manners
2. Drinks at a Chinese table
3. Eating at a Chinese table
4. Rules and conventions relating to chopsticks
5. Seating arrangements for a Chinese banquet

References for Further Discussion

1. Most table manners in China are similar to in the West. Don't be deceived by what you might see in a local restaurant on the streets. Chinese manners don't consist of slurping food down as quickly as possible, and shouting loudly!

A. Consider Others

1) When helping yourself to the dishes, you should take food first from the plates in front of you rather than those in the middle of the table or in front of others. It's bad manners to use your chopsticks to burrow through the food and "dig for treasure" and keep your eyes glued to the plates. 2) When finding your favorite dish, you should not gobble it up as quickly as possible or put the plate in front of yourself and proceed to eat like a horse. You should consider others at the table. If there is not much left on a plate and you want to finish it, you should consult others. If they say they don't want any more, then you can proceed to eat. 3) Concentrate on the meal and your companions. Watching television, using your phone, or carrying on some other activities while having a meal is considered a bad habit. 4) You should try to refill your bowl with rice yourself and take the initiative to fill the bowls of elders with rice and food from the dishes. If elders fill your bowl or add food to your bowl, you should express your thanks.

B. "Thank you" Gesture

1) Tea usually is served as soon as you have a seat in a restaurant. A waiter/waitress serves you tea while you read the menu and decide what to order. The tea pot is left with you on the table after everyone around the table's cup is filled with tea. Guests then serve themselves. 2) When someone pours tea into your cup, you can tap the table with your first two fingers two or three times, showing thanks to the pourer for the service and of being enough tea. The pourer will stop pouring when seeing the gesture.

2. There are several kinds of drinks at a Chinese table such as wine, alcohol, but more tea is a more common drink. 1) The host should always make sure everyone's cups are not empty for long. One should not pour for oneself. It would be good to offer to pour drink for the person sitting next to you and he/she will in turn pour drink for you. 2) Make sure the spout of the teapot is not facing anyone; it is impolite to set the teapot down where the spout is facing towards somebody. The spout should always be directed to where nobody is sitting, usually just outward from the table. 3) When people wish to clink

drinks together in the form of a cheer, it is important to observe that younger members should clink the rim of their glass below the rim of an elder's to show respect.

Strong alcohol, called *baijiu*, is often served throughout the meal; and it is customary for the hosts/hostesses to insist that guests drink to "show friendship." If the guests prefer not to drink, they may say, "I'm unable to drink, but thank you." The host may continue to insist that the guests drink, and the guests may likewise continue to insist upon being "unable" to drink. The host's insistence is to show generosity. Therefore, refusal by the guests should be made with utmost politeness. Beware: If a guest drinks alcohol with a subordinate at the table, the guest will be expected (if not forced) to drink a glass of the same alcohol with each superior at that table, and possibly at other tables too—if the guest has not passed out yet.

3. 1) Pick the food on the dish that is at the top and nearest to you in distance. Never rummage through the dish or pick from the far side for your favorite food. 2) In general, more conservative Chinese frown upon the practice of picking more than one or two bites of food in your bowl or serving plate as if you were eating in the Western way. 3) If both a serving bowl—separate from rice bowl—and plate are provided, never put any food items to be eaten onto the serving plate. This rule may be relaxed for foreigners. 4) If a dish is soupy, pull the serving bowl near the serving dish and reduce the distance the chopsticks need carrying the food. Spilling plenty of sauce on the table is a major faux pas. 5) When eating food that contains bones, it is customary that the bones be spat out onto the table to the right of the dining plate in a neat pile. Spitting onto the floor is almost never acceptable. 6) Talking with a full mouth, eating with the elbows on the table and tasting from a table guest's plate is also not allowed.

4. 1) Chopsticks should always be held correctly, i. e. between the thumb and first two fingers of the right hand. 2) When not in use, chopsticks must always be placed neatly on the table with two sticks lying tidily next to each other at both ends. Failure to do so is evocative of the way the dead would be placed in a coffin before the funeral. 3) Never point the chopsticks at another person. This amounts to insulting that person. 4) Never wave your chopsticks around as if they were an extension of your hand gestures. 5) Never bang chopsticks like drumsticks. This is akin to telling others at the table you are a beggar. 6) Never use chopsticks to move bowls or plates. 7) Never suck the chopsticks. 8) Decide what to pick up before reaching with chopsticks, instead of hovering them over or rummaging through dishes. 9) To keep chopsticks off the table, they can be rested horizontally on one's plate or bowl; a chopstick rest (commonly found in restaurants) can also be used. 10) When picking up a piece of food, never use the tips of your chopsticks to poke through the food as with a fork; exceptions include tearing apart larger items such as vegetables. 11) Never stab chopsticks vertically into a bowl of rice, as this resembles incense sticks used at temples to pay respects to the deceased.

5. The seating arrangement is probably the most important part of Chinese dining

etiquette. Dining etiquette in ancient times was enacted according to a four-tier social strata: i) the imperial court, ii) local authorities, iii) trade associations and iv) farmers and workers. The respect structure in modern dining etiquette has been simplified to: i) master of the banquet and ii) guests.

1) Seat of Honor: The seat of honor, reserved for the master of the banquet or the guest with highest status, is the one in the center facing east or facing the entrance. Those of higher position sit closer to the master of the banquet. The guests of lowest position sit furthest from the seat of honor. When a family holds a banquet, the seat of honor is for the guest with the highest status and the head of the house takes the least prominent seat.

2) Round Table: If round tables are used, the seat facing the entrance is the seat of honor. The seats on the left hand side of the seat of honor are second, fourth, sixth, etc. in importance, while those on the right are the third, fifth, seventh and so on in importance, until they join together.

3) Square Table: In ancient times there was a piece of furniture known as an Eight Immortals table, a big square table with benches for two people on each side. If there was a seat facing the entrance, then the right hand seat when facing the entrance was for the guest of honor. If there was no seat facing the entrance door (presumably if the meal was outside or there were two or more doors of equal importance), then the right hand seat when facing east was the seat of honor. The seats on the left hand side of the seat of honor were, in order of importance, second, fourth, sixth and eighth and those on the right were third, fifth and seventh.

4) In Grand Banquet: In a grand banquet of many tables, the table of honor is the one furthest from the entrance (or facing east in the event of no clear main entrance). The tables on the left hand side of the tables of honor are, in order of importance, second, fourth, sixth and so on, and those on the right are third, fifth and seventh. Guests are seated according to their status and degree of relationship to the master of the banquet.

Unit 7

Key Points

Learning Targets

- To *make a speech* with a given topic
- To *make a presentation* based on the given reading materials
- To learn about the academic terms of urology in clinical diagnostic conversation

Learning Focus

- How to solicit comments and limit the speech time of speakers at an international academic conference

Cultural Points

- Chinese tea culture

✓音、视频资源
✓参考译文
✓参考答案
✓学术探讨

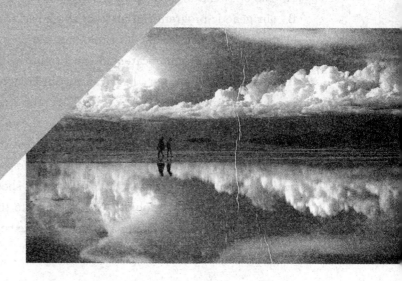

Part I   Listening Comprehension

Video 1

Cancer Cure

Exercise I   Choose correct answers to the following questions.

1. The speaker compared the bacteria in our body with stars in our galaxy because _____ .

   A. the bacteria in our body can grow and explode like stars in our galaxy

   B. there are a great number of bacteria in our body

   C. scientists can observe bacteria in our body as they observe stars in the universe

   D. stars in our galaxy may have an effect on the bacteria in our body

2. According to the speech, the growing colony of bacteria in the film is as wide as _____ .

   A. a human liver   B. a human tooth

   C. a human hair   D. a human cell

3. The speaker can program bacteria to detect and treat cancer because _____ .

   A. bacteria tend to develop in those tumors

   B. our genetic program can instruct these bacteria to produce small molecules

   C. those bacteria look like an exploding star

   D. bacteria can communicate and synchronize with each other

4. According to the speaker, liver cancer can be detected by _____ of your urine.

   A. the temperature   B. the smell

   C. the amount   D. the color

5. How the programmed bacteria are used to treat cancer?

   A. Programmed bacteria may produce some therapeutic molecules to kill the tumors.

   B. Programmed bacteria will be instructed to shoot at the tumor areas.

   C. The health benefit probiotics will transform the tumors into benign ones.

   D. Those programmed bacteria can change the color of the tumors.

Exercise II   Watch the video and decide whether the following statements are true (T) or false (F).

6. To program the bacteria is to change the DNA inside of them so that these bacteria can help us detect and treat tumors.

7. Genetic program instructs the bacteria to produce large molecules and tell other bacteria when to turn on and off.

8. The genetic program depends on the so-called quorum sensing.

9. Tumors are not safe for those probiotics because of the immune system.

10. Liver cancer can also be detected by other means with ease.

Video 2 ▌▌▌▌

Medical Inventions

Exercise I   Choose correct answers to the following questions.

1. How long does it take for a patient to recognize the symptoms of a heart attack?
   A. 3 minutes   B. 43 seconds
   C. 3 hours   D. one day

2. How many people will suffer from an everlasting damage to their heart in America annually?
   A. 600,000   B. 300,000
   C. 1. 2 million   D. 900,000

3. According to the speech, why do men usually refuse to admit the symptoms of a heart attack?
   A. Because men are afraid of these symptoms.
   B. Because men are brave.
   C. Because these symptoms are not serious.
   D. Becausemen don't feel such symptoms.

4. What is a certain sign of a heart attack?
   A. A higher blood pressure
   B. An increase of one part of ST segment
   C. An increase of basic body temperature
   D. A severe headache or chest pain

5. The FDA won't allow us to use the device on people unless _____.
   A. we sell the device to other countries

B. the device can save the life of enough people

C. the device can beep or vibrate

D. we prove the device effective and reliable enough

Exercise Ⅱ   Watch the video and decide whether the following statements are true (T) or false (F).

6. People with silent ischemia will spend less time recognizing the symptoms of a heart attack.

7. Every year, there are 1. 2 million Americans who suffer from a heart attack.

8. Approximately 75 percent of patients in America never have any symptoms.

9. Diabetics and elderly women are at a higher risk of a heart attack.

10. Pigs are the best experimental subject for our device.

Listening 1

To Cure Alzheimer's

Exercise Ⅰ   Choose correct answers to the following questions.

1. What did Alois find in Auguste's brain?

A. He found many worms in her brain.

B. He found strange plaques and tangles in her brain.

C. He found many blood clots in her brain.

D. He found a tumor in her brain.

2. How many people will be affected by Alzheimer's by 2050?

A. 85 million   B. 40 million

C. 150 million   D. 114 million

3. According to the speech, why did the government pay little attention to Alzheimer's these years?

A. Because of the lack of awareness.

B. Because it is difficult to cure Alzheimer's.

C. Because curing Alzheimer's will cost a lot of money.

D. Because the government knew that Alzheimer's couldn't be prevented, cured or even slowed down.

4. According to the speaker, which one is NOT the harmfulness of Alzheimer's?

A. Alzheimer's will lead to severe loss of one's memory.

B. Alzheimer's can result in some disorders in one's mind.

C. Alzheimer's may shorten one's life expectancy.

D. Alzheimer's will cause high blood pressure or diabetes.

5. Which statement is true according to the speech?

A. Strictly speaking, Alzheimer's is not a disease because it is incurable.

B. Nowadays we have made much progress in treating Alzheimer's after so many years.

C. Alzheimer's may affect more women than men.

D. Even some scientists mistakenly confused Alzheimer's with the process of aging.

Exercise Ⅱ Listen to the material and decide whether the following statements are true (T) or false (F).

6. The disease was named after Alzheimer because he was the first patient who was diagnosed with such a disease.

7. Alzheimer's has been the most expensive disease and biggest medical challenge nowadays.

8. At present, we can't cure Alzheimer's, but we can prevent it before it happens.

9. According to the speech, every year, cancers cause more deaths than Alzheimer's.

10. Usually, Alzheimer's can cause some mental problems, but it is not fatal.

Listening 2 ||||

Long-term Delivery of Monoclonal Antibodies with Potent Neutralizing Activity against a Broad Range of HIV Isolates

Exercise Ⅰ Listen to the material and decide whether the following statements are true (T) or false (F).

1. The first person asking questions was wondering as the speaker has had serum from all the other monkeys that have anti-drug antibodies, if that could be a method of trying to assess whether he has cured the monkey or not.

2. The FDA may raise the question whether there are ways to remove the antibodies or stop it in human testing if problems do develop.

3. The speaker has done muscle biopsies in some of these monkeys, and marked the area of inoculation.

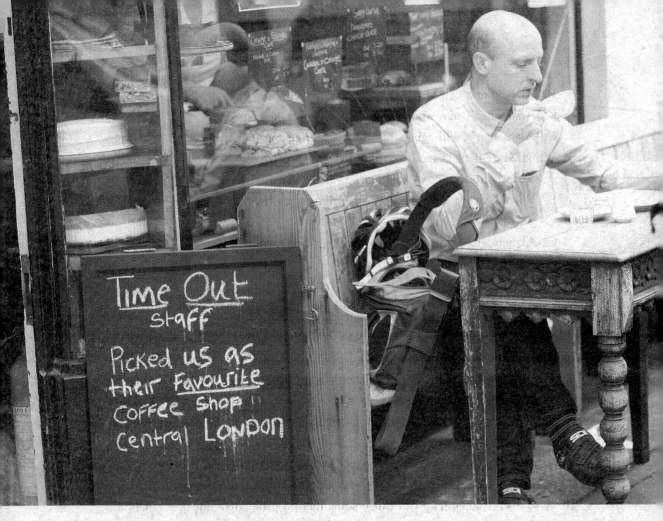

4. Since it is hard to imagine being able to deliver enough of the anti-idio type antibodies to totally remove what's there, it's not an approach that could be considered.

5. The speaker said they chose shiv-ad8 for two reasons. First, it was a cloned virus. Second, Malcolm's data indicated there was a quite consistent viral load set point.

6. Before the speaker selected the antibodies he was going to use, he checked to make sure they had good neutralizing activity against the strain he was using.

7. If they didn't transfer virus with the adoptive transfer, they needn't get more animals and broad assays many years.

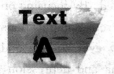
Text
A

More than 100 Million Americans Have Diabetes or Prediabetes
— Lifestyle Changes Can Prevent Full-blown Disease

Robert Preidt

More than 100 million U. S. adults have diabetes or prediabetes, health officials say.

As of 2015, more than 9 percent of the population—30. 3 million—had diabetes. Another 84. 1 million had prediabetes, the U. S. Centers for Disease Control and Prevention reported Tuesday.

People with prediabetes have elevated blood sugar levels, but not so high that they have full-blown diabetes, which requires medication or insulin injections. With exercise and a healthy diet, prediabetics can halve their risk of developing type 2 diabetes, the CDC noted.

However, awareness levels remain too low. The new report found that nearly 1 in 4 adults with diabetes didn't even know they had the disease, and less than 12 percent with prediabetes knew they had that condition. If not treated, prediabetes often leads to type 2 diabetes within five years, the CDC said. "More than a third of U. S. adults have prediabetes, and the majority don't know it," CDC Director Dr. Brenda Fitzgerald said. "Now, more than ever, we must step up our efforts to reduce the burden of this serious disease," she said in a government news release.

According to the report, the rate of new diabetes cases remains steady: 1. 5 million new cases were diagnosed among people 18 and older in 2015. Incidence rose with age. Four percent of adults ages 18 to 44 had diagnosed diabetes, compared with 17 percent of people 45 to 64, and one-quarter of folks 65 and older.

Dr. Minisha Sood is an endocrinologist at Lenox Hill Hospital in New York City. "It is reassuring that the rate of increase in diabetes cases has slowed, but we should not reduce our vigilance when it comes to optimizing metabolic health for Americans," Sood said. "Prevention is key to avoid the development of the condition in the first place. Optimal nutrition education and access to good nutrition is critical to our success as a medical community in the battle to prevent diabetes in the U. S. ," Sood added. By focusing on prevention, it may be possible to avoid the numerous complications of diabetes and obesity, which include not only eye, kidney and nerve problems but also dental disease, dementia and depression, Sood said.

Some of the report highlights: Rates of diagnosed diabetes were higher for American Indians/Alaska Natives (15 percent), blacks (nearly 13 percent), and Hispanics (12 percent) than for Asians (8 percent) and whites (7. 4 percent). Prevalence also differed by education. The highest rate—nearly 13 percent—was among those with less than a high school education. Adults with more than a high school education had the lowest rate—a little over 7 percent. By U. S. region, the South and Appalachia had the highest rates of diagnosed diabetes and new diabetes cases. Rates of prediabetes were higher among men (nearly 37 percent) than among women (29 percent). Diabetes is the seventh leading cause of death in the United States.

Certain trends stand out in this report, said Dr. Howard Selinger, chair of family medicine at Quinnipiac University in North Haven, Conn. "The highest incidence among prediabetes and diabetes occurs in those individuals with lower income, less education and to a large degree who live in rural areas," he said. Type 2 diabetes is overwhelmingly more prevalent than type 1 diabetes, which occurs earlier in life and has a stronger genetic predisposition, Selinger noted. Type 2 tends to be lifestyle-related. The nation could make a tremendous difference in the prevalence of diabetes and its health complications by seriously promoting a healthier diet, facilitating a more active lifestyle and providing access to quality preventive and primary health care for those most in need, he said.

Ann Albright of the CDC agreed that more needs to be done to halt diabetes. "Consistent with previous trends, our research shows that diabetes cases are still increasing, although not as quickly as in previous years," said Albright, director of CDC's division of diabetes

医学英语学术交流教程

translation.

"By addressing diabetes, we limit other health problems such as heart disease, stroke, nerve and kidney diseases, and vision loss," she said.

(737 words)

※ Source: U. S. Centers for Disease Control and Prevention, July 18, 2017; Minisha Sood, M. D., endocrinologist, Lenox Hill Hospital, New York City; Howard Selinger, M. D., chair, family medicine, Frank H. Netter M. D. School of Medicine, Quinnipiac University, North Haven, Conn.

Vocabulary

halve	[hɑːv]	vt.	二等分，减半
release	[rɪˈliːs]	n.	释放，发表（消息），公布
endocrinologist	[ˌendəʊkraɪˈnɒlədʒɪst]	n.	内分泌学家
optimize	[ˈɒptɪmaɪz]	vt.	使最优化；使发挥最大效用
dementia	[dɪˈmenʃɪə]	n.	痴呆，智力衰退
overwhelmingly	[ˌəʊvəˈwelmɪŋlɪ]	adv.	势不可挡地，极大地
predisposition	[priːˌdɪspəˈzɪʃən]	n.	倾向，素因，素质，体质
facilitate	[fəˈsɪlɪteɪt]	vt.	使变容易，使便利，促进

Read the text and decide whether the following statements are true (T) or false (F).

1. Nearly half of adults with diabetes in US are unaware of their condition.
2. Nowadays the increase rate of diabetes cases is quicker than ever before.
3. The incidences of diabetes among Hispanics and whites are higher than that of the Asians.
4. The older you are, the more likely you may have diabetes.
5. Some heart diseases, mental diseases, eye problems and even dental problems are related to diabetes.

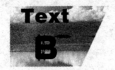

Social Sciences and Malnutrition

Igor de Garine

Malnutrition is a complex topic and implies collaboration between the biological and the human sciences. If we accept the yardsticks provided by modern nutritional science, biologists have at their disposal techniques that will rapidly provide objective measurements to assess the state of nutrition of the various categories of individuals in a population. It is possible to determine who is suffering from malnutrition, but identifying the factors responsible for it is another problem.

The human being is an omnivorous consumer whose feeding behavior is largely conditioned by his or her culture. Both material and nonmaterial aspects of culture should be taken into account in order to understand the causes of malnutrition. But which ones? Obviously those directly related to the diet, such as food production, should be considered, but religious beliefs, for instance, can also have an impact. The weight of the factors involved may vary according to the society considered. This is why the holistic approach of the anthropologist, sifting through the various domains of culture, may reveal the hierarchy of causes.

Which aspects should be analyzed? In the field of material culture, the following: food production, preservation, storage, commercialization, and technology; cooking and consumption of foods and liquids; and also family budgets, with special reference to food.

In nonmaterial culture, knowledge about local animals and plants, social and religious organizations in relation to food production and consumption, social and religious rituals involving food, prestige in relation to food (food as a link, food as a marker, food and body shape), knowledge in relation to nutrition and health, and opinions and attitudes (preferences and rejections) in relation to food should be analyzed.

Psychosocial aspects related to food may also be examined: the learning process (through family, peers, or the media) and the psychopathological aspects related to food (bulimia and anorexia).

However, in the past, food-consumption surveys by the weighing method, combined with ethnographic studies on food, have given good results in organizing applied nutrition programs. They oblige the investigators to have close contact with the population and gain some knowledge of domestic life, which may be very useful in understanding the causes of malnutrition and elaborating a pertinent program.

Today, these techniques have been discarded as expensive, time-consuming, and concerning only small samples. It can be argued that these detailed studies carried out on representative samples can be a preliminary stage allowing the organization of a more extensive survey, using lighter sociological techniques and including a statistically significant sample. A subtle analysis of locally available wild food allows the specific causes of malnutrition to be detected and pertinent methods to fight them to be found. There is always something to be done.

In the past, action programs were aimed mostly at fighting the lack of food and, to a certain extent, inadequate amounts of nutrients in the diet.

Today a major problem has appeared: managing food abundance in wealthy societies. Technological advances have made it possible to consume any kind of food in any quantity at any time of the year in any part of the world, provided the potential consumers can pay for it. The result is a tendency to overeat and to adopt a diet in which fats, sugar, and animal proteins dominate. At the same time, energy expenditure is low. The outcome is obesity and the occurrence of a whole range of physical ailments such as cardiovascular disease and diabetes. Particular mention should be made of obesity among the poor, due mainly to the excess consumption of cheap carbohydrates.

The physical ideal is a slim body, which is very difficult indeed to obtain. Beliefs in food pollution and the aggression of daily life, among other factors, result in psychopathological diseases, such as anorexia nervosa and bulimia. This implies a need for the increased participation of psychology specialists to solve the problem of malnutrition, which today is as much dependent on the personal history of individuals as on the constraints of their culture, which has offered them, from the onset of their life, a broad choice of food. In practice, the result is that to determine features justifying public health measures. It is necessary to consider very large samples and resort to sociological approaches.

A new aspect should be mentioned: in the aggressive and competitive Western world, as well as in insecure acculturating groups, foods and drinks appear to be used as stress relievers. In this respect alcoholism is becoming, at the global level, an important factor in malnutrition.

In preindustrial societies, traditional knowledge is not necessarily in line with scientific nutrition principles. Malnutrition is seldom perceived and is not necessarily traced to locally available wild food but may be attributed to magical practices or to the breaking of a taboo. Very little is known about nutritional requirements. For example, the specific needs of weanling children are rarely evaluated efficiently. The supplementation of their diet may be merely quantitative, and animal-protein foods may be prohibited for fear of gastric disorders or magical influences.

On specific issues, social scientists can help detect the causes of malnutrition and suggest measures to improve the situation. They can also help motivate the policymakers. In general terms, since there is no innate nutritional wisdom, adequate nutrition principles have to be learned. Social scientists can help in any type of society to develop educational programs to impart sound nutritional knowledge at an early age. This may allow people to react critically to the flux of unreliable nutritional information to which they are constantly exposed and could potentially lead to rational feeding behavior.

Finally, in the field of fundamental research, anthropologists, through their meticulous approach to humans in their normal environment and their interest in societies outside the scope of the modern Western world, may still allow original hypotheses to be developed in the field of nutrition, about which there is still so much to learn.

(975 words)

※ The text is extracted from the keynote address from the First World Congress on Public Health Nutrition. The author is affiliated with the Centre National de la Recherche Scientifique (CNRS), France.

Part Ⅲ　Oral Practice

Practice 1 ▮▮▮▮
Clinical Inquiry—Department of Urology

 Brainstorming

A. Try to brainstorm as many words and phrases which are relevant to the urinary system or urology department as possible.

B. The following are for your reference. Match the medical terms with their Chinese equivalent.

urology	尿痛
urinary frequency	早泄
computed tomography（CT）	血尿
odynuria	泌尿外科学
urgent urination	肾绞痛
interrupted urination	尿频
magnetic resonance imaging（MRI）	膀胱疼痛
haematuria	计算机断层摄影
nephric colic	勃起功能障碍
bladder pain	泌尿系平片
prostatodynia	血精
testalgia	尿液分析
erectile disfunction（ED）	尿急
premature ejaculation	镜检
hematospermia	肾功能检查
urine analysis	尿中断
polyuria	肿瘤标志物检查
test under microscope	静脉尿路造影
renal function	多尿
tumor markers examination	尿道膀胱造影
plain film of the urinary system（KUB）	睾丸痛

intravenous urography（IVU）		磁共振成像扫描
urethrocystography		肾图
radioisotope examination		腔道泌尿外科学
nephrogram		前列腺痛
endourology		放射性同位素检查肾图

Dialogue：A Patient's Complaints and Symptoms of Disorders in the Urinary System

Study and simulate the following sample dialogue，pay special attention to the way the patient offers his main complaints. Some of the words and expressions that you've come up with in the previous part may be of help.

pyuria	[paɪˈjuərɪə]	n.	脓尿
incontinence	[ɪnˈkɒntɪnəns]	n.	尿失禁
urgency	[ˈɜːdʒənsɪ]	n.	尿急
odynuria	[ɒdɪnˈjuərɪə]	n.	尿痛
polyuria	[ˈpɒlɪˈjərɪə]	n.	多尿
dysuresia	[diːˈʃuəzə]	n.	排尿困难
frequency	[ˈfriːkwənsɪ]	n.	尿频
haematuria	[heməˈtjuərɪə]	n.	血尿
nephric colic	[ˈnefrɪk ˈkɒlɪk]	n.	肾绞痛
urinalysis	[ˌjuərɪˈnælɪsɪs]	n.	尿液分析
three-glass test			尿三杯检查
urine examination of castoff cells			尿脱落细胞检查

Sample Dialogue

Patient：Well，doc，I have been feeling so poorly recently. Something must be wrong with my making water.

Doctor：What do you mean by that? Are you having any situation with your urinary system? I mean waterworks.

Patient：Waterworks? Yes，it seems that I do have to go for a pee more often than I used to.

Doctor：Can you describe that in more detail? Say，when did it start? What's the frequency? Or how often is that?

Patient：It's sometimes every hour or even more often，but you know，it depends. So is it so-called polyuria? Or frequent micturition? I've been googling such things these days.

Doctor: Don't be anxious. We are not there yet to jump to early conclusions.

Patient: OK. Go on. I'm all ears.

Doctor: Do you have to get up to pee at night recently?

Patient: Yes. It's two or three times, sort of.

Doctor: You feel any pain when you pass water?

Patient: Yes, at first it only came and went when I'm passing water. Gradually, I have it all the time. It worsens at times. It seems to come over me in waves, but mostly it's there all the time now.

Doctor: Could you please describe what the pain feels like? It's stabbing? Or colicky? Burning?

Patient: It's burning, and sometimes I can feel a knife-like pain even.

Doctor: Can you point out the painful area?

Patient: It's here, the lower abdomen. Yeah, right here.

Doctor: I'd like to feel your abdomen. Put your arms down by your side and let your tummy or stomach relax, ... that's it. Are there any places that are tender or painful? Now I want to check your liver and spleen, so take deep breath in, hold it, ... fine. Nothing special. OK, we're almost done. Do you have any trouble getting started?

Patient: No, not really.

Doctor: Do you have urgency, I mean, urgent urination? Or interrupted urination?

Patient: No, never.

Doctor: Do you ever lose control of your bladder? Any leaking or dribbling?

Patient: Well, perhaps a little dribbling from time to time.

Doctor: What about pyuria and haematuria? I mean, have you ever passed blood in the urine?

Patient: No, never.

Doctor: OK. Considering your situation, I expect you to have some examination and tests, including a urinalysis and urine castoff cells examination, a three-glass test and a renal function test, which hopefully can give us a big picture of your problem and your situation will be then scientifically diagnosed.

Patient: OK, then, is it serious? I'm very nervous and ...

Doctor: Please don't be. You must have a bee in your head but it's not necessary. Let's wait for the results firstly. OK?

Patient: OK, I'm overreacted actually.

Doctor: Very well, and I'll make you those appointments as soon as possible ...

Activities and Role-play (inviting students to improvise and act it out)

Practice 2

International Conference
—Soliciting Comments and Limiting Time

 Useful Expressions for Soliciting Comments

1. It's a very good/important/excellent/interesting/difficult/complicated research. Any questions or comments for Dr. Williams?

2. Does everyone already have the handout for reference? OK, it's time for discussion, do you have any questions?

3. May I have your attention please? Any more/further questions or comments for Dr. Green?

4. Any objection to the application of the method provided by Dr. Zhuang?

5. It's appreciated if you could have questions or comments on my work.

6. It'll be quite a privilege for you to comment on my research.

7. Are there any further questions? OK, let's have the following presentation from the next speaker.

 Useful Expressions for Limiting Time

1. Dr. Jordan, thanks for asking, but I'm sorry, we do have to move on; we are running short of time.

2. Ladies and gentlemen, the schedule is quite/very/rather tight. So we haven't any time for more discussion, and we must go on to the next paper.

3. There are some basic rules to be reaffirmed. At the end of each presentation, there will be 5 minutes for discussion before we move on to the next speaker. And if the discussion time is not enough for you and you still have other questions or comments, we will have an open discussion on any of the papers presented at the end of the session.

4. Let's turn/move on to the next problem/subject of the study after the stretch.

5. I think that'll be the last/final question before we move on to the next speaker.

6. I am afraid I won't have time to cover everything of my presentation.

7. Time is limited; I will go through over the next three points very briefly.

8. Due to the limited time, please contemplate and organize your thoughts carefully before raising your questions. Thanks for cooperation.

9. To make good use of the limited time, please simplify your questions and comments which are expected to be no more than two aspects.

Practice 3 ||||

Oral English for Culture and on Social Occasions —Tea Culture

Useful Words and Phrases

1. Tea drinking is a very sophisticated pastime instead of an action to simply quench one's thirst.

2. In ancient China, scholars would use fine cups to drink tea and they call it "to savor" in such graceful ambiences as "spring water runs on marbles", "in a monastery in misty spring", "bamboos in the moonlight" and "in the woods during sunset".

3. Fine people use different kinds of exquisite tea sets but the most popular ones are the pots made in Yixing.

4. There are several categories of tea, including red tea, green tea, Oolong tea and Pu'er tea.

5. Pu'er tea contains a kind of healthy fungus, which will ferment on its own after the tea is long processed. This is why expensive Pu'er tea is always quite old.

6. Tea drinking can help a person achieve an elevated state of mind, which is said to be originally the monks' pursuit of tranquility and later imitated by ordinary people as an elegant pastime.

7. Tea houses and tea parties are now popular in both vulgar life and the business world. When in official circle, tea drinking even represents thriftiness and cleanliness.

8. A cup of tea, not only serves social and economic purposes, but also political as well. No wonder tea is always with food in Chinese culture.

9. Compared with drinking coffee, it's a lot more sophisticated to drink tea, which is deeply rooted in the traditional Chinese culture.

10. Tea drinking can immerse you in the traditions, and you can reach a state of tranquility and harmony.

Activities and Role-play (inviting students to improvise and act it out)

Topics for Further Discussion

1. Tea and China
2. Tea or coffee
3. Fashion of tea drinking
4. Tea and Chinese culture
5. Art of teaism

References for Further Discussion

Tea Culture in China (1)

The Chinese people, in their drinking of tea, place much significance on the act of "savoring". "Savoring tea" is not only a way to discern good tea from mediocre tea, but also how people take delight in their reverie and in tea-drinking itself. Snatching a bit of leisure from a busy schedule, making a kettle of strong tea, securing a serene space, and serving and drinking tea by yourself can help banish fatigue and frustration, improve your thinking ability and inspire you with enthusiasm. You may also imbibe it slowly in small sips to appreciate the subtle allure of tea-drinking, until your spirits soar up and up into a sublime aesthetic realm. Buildings, gardens, ornaments and tea sets are the elements that form the ambience for savoring tea. A tranquil, refreshing, comfortable and neat locale is certainly desirable for drinking tea. Chinese gardens are well known in the world and beautiful Chinese landscapes are too numerous to count. Teahouses tucked away in gardens and nestled beside the natural beauty of mountains and rivers are enchanting places of repose for people to rest and recreate themselves.

China is a country with a time-honored civilization and a land of ceremony and decorum. Whenever guests visit, it is necessary to make and serve tea to them. Before serving tea, you may ask them for their preferences as to what kind of tea they fancy and serve them the tea in the most appropriate teacups. In the course of serving tea, the host should take careful note of how much water is remaining in the cups and in the kettle. Usually, if the tea is made in a teacup, boiling water should be added after half of the cup has been consumed; and thus the cup is kept filled so that the tea retains the same bouquet and remains pleasantly warm throughout the entire course of tea-drinking. Snacks, sweets and other dishes may be served at tea time to complement the fragrance of the tea and to allay one's hunger.

Tea Culture in China (2)

There are three most famous drinks in the world. They are tea, coffee and cocoa. China is the homeland of tea which has become the national drink. Referring to Chinese tea culture, it has several thousand years of history and can be traced back to the ancient times. Then it was flourished in the Tang Dynasty and the Song Dynasty.

In China, the main varieties of tea are green tea, black tea, Oolong tea, scented tea, white tea, yellow tea and dark tea. We make different tea in different particular ways. Over the centuries, China developed an extraordinary tea culture, comparable with the coffee culture of the West.

Tea has not only a good flavor but also benefit to our body, so it is loved by many people home and abroad. Different kinds of tea have different function which makes a contribution to our health. For example, the national drink of China-green tea, can dispel the effects of alcohol, refresh yourself and whiten your skin. The second largest kind of tea-black tea, can warm your stomach, be good for your heart and make your bones stronger. Dark tea can refresh you in the morning, reduce your blood press and help lose weight. Oolong Tea is good for your body building and dieting. In all, tea has great medicinal value: anti-cancer, lowering blood pressure, improving eyesight and restraining disease, reducing stress and so on. Tea culture and its development reflect not only diet culture, but also Chinese spiritual features. Tea culture plays an indispensable role in promoting the international cultural exchange between China and other countries, enriching Chinese cultural life and promoting Chinese spiritual civilization construction.

In conclusion, tea culture is one of the essences of Chinese culture in the history. The spirit of tea permeates the court and society, into the Chinese poetry, painting, calligraphy, religion, and medicine. For thousands of years China has not only accumulated a great deal about tea cultivation, production of material culture, but also accumulated rich spirit of the tea culture, which is unique to China's tea culture.

Unit 8

Key Points

Learning Targets
- To practice *comprehensive listening skills*
- To make comments on peers' presentations
- To learn about the academic terms used in operating rooms

Learning Focus
- How to deliver an acceptant speech and words of congratulations at an international academic conference

Cultural Points
- Buddhism in China

✓音、视频资源
✓参考译文
✓参考答案
✓学术探讨

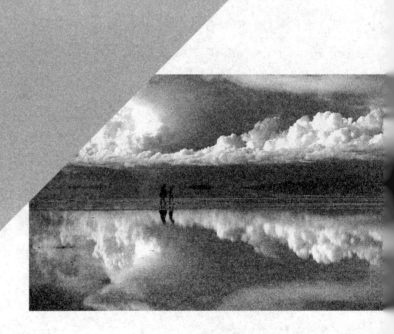

Video 1 ||||
Speech at the Sixty-eighth World Health Assembly

Exercise I Choose correct answers to the following questions.

1. According to the speech, where is WHO NOT responding at present?
   A. South Africa   B. Liberia   C. Nepal   D. Sierra Leone

2. On May 9th, WHO declared that the Ebola outbreak _____ in Liberia.
   A. started   B. was put out   C. spread wider   D. became less severe

3. The Ebola outbreak has stimulated WHO to reform faster, coping first with _____.
   A. wide-spread infectious diseases
   B. medical services in catastrophes
   C. the low efficiency of WHO resource management
   D. changes in WHO emergency operations.

4. The world expects from WHO _____.
   A. streamlined administrative procedures that support stronger action
   B. effective financial coordination with others
   C. clear lines of command and control
   D. speedy community engagement and better communications

5. Which is NOT an aim of Dr. Chan's newly-created programme?
   A. Speed   B. Performance benchmarks
   C. Rapid impact   D. Flexibility

Exercise II Watch the video and decide whether the following statements are true (T) or false (F).

6. With a history of over 70 years, WHO still hasn't got the world well prepared for an outbreak so widespread, severe, sustained and complex like Ebola.

7. President Ellen Johnson Sirleaf played an important role in the fight with Ebola crisis.

8. Fighting alone with various crisis and catastrophes, WHO is now overwhelmed.

9. After the battle with Ebola, WHO realized the urgent need of reform.

10. To command and control better, Dr. Chan has six Regional Directors to advise and make minor decisions for her.

Video 2

How Does Nervous System Work?

Exercise I Crossword the following words based on what you've understood. You may refer to the hints in the Across-Down region below if necessary.

| convert | transmit | recoil | gate | thermal |
| pore | gradient | overshoot | depolarization | synapse |

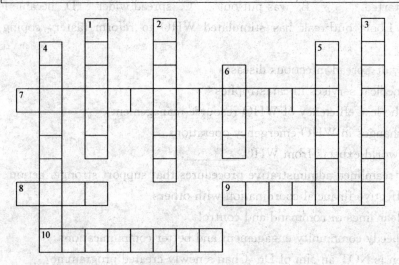

ACROSS

7. elimination of polarization

8. one of the very small holes in cell membrane that element particles can pass or in your skin that sweat can pass through

9. to change or make sth change from one form, purpose, system, etc. to another

DOWN

1. to move your body quickly away from sb/sth because you find them or it frightening or unpleasant with strong dislike or fear

2. relating to or caused by heat or by changes in temperature

3. the rate at which concentration, temperature, pressure, etc. changes,

10. to send an electronic signal, radio or television broadcast, etc

or increases and decreases, between one region and another

4. to go futher than the place one intended to stop or turn

5. one of the points in the nervous system at which a signal passes from one nerve cell to another

6. to switch electronic waves, electronic signals, and electrical power

Exercise II Fill in the blanks with the original words and phrases or with expressions which have the same or the closest meaning.

11. Nerves have a much more complex job in the body. They are not just wires, but the cells that are the sensors, detectors of the _____ and internal world, the transducers that convert information to electrical _____, the wires that _____ these impulses, the transistors that _____ the information and turn up or down the volume and finally, the _____ that take the information and cause it to have an effect on other organs.

12. Each of those neurons is highly _____ to carry nerve impulses, their form of _____, in response to only one kind of stimulus, and in only one direction.

13. The inside of a nerve is a fluid that is very rich in the ion _____. It is 20 times higher than in the fluid outside the nerve while that outside fluid has 10 times more _____ than the inside of a nerve.

14. After depolarization, _____ pump the sodium back out of the nerve and the potassium back into the nerve, restoring the nerve to its _____.

15. It is here, in this _____, that the neuron's electrical information can be modulated, _____, blocked altogether or translated to another informational process.

Listening 1 ‖‖‖
Surgery's Past, Present and Robotic Future

Exercise I Take notes and fill in the blanks in the following sentences.

A. Until anesthesia, the absence of 1. _____. With the demonstration of the

Morton Ether Inhaler at the Mass. General in 1847, a whole new era of surgery was ushered in. Anesthesia gave 2. _____ the freedom to 3. _____. Anesthesia gave them the freedom to 4. _____, to start to delve deeper into the body. This was truly a 5. _____ in surgery.

B. After these very long, 6. _____ operations, attempting to cure things they'd never been able to touch before, the patients died. They died of 7. _____. Surgery didn't hurt anymore, but it killed you pretty quickly. And infection would continue to claim a 8. _____ of surgical patients until the next big revolution in surgery, which was 9. _____.

C. With the patient 10. _____ to pain, and a 11. _____ operating field all bets were off, the sky was the limit. You could now start doing surgery everywhere, on the gut, on the 12. _____, on the heart, on the brain. 13. _____: you could take an 14. _____ out of one person, you could put it in another person, and it would work.

D. "Well, can we do these same surgeries but through little 15. _____?" 16. _____ is doing this kind of surgery: surgery with long 17. _____ through small incisions. And it really changed the landscape of surgery. Some of the tools for this have been around for a hundred years, but it had only been used as a 18. _____ technique until the 1980s.

Listing 2 |||||

Color-coded Surgery

Exercise I   Take notes and fill in the blanks in the following sentences.

A. In surgery, it's important to know what to 1. _____. But equally important is to 2. _____ things that are important for 3. _____. So it's very important to avoid inadvertent 4. _____. And what I'm talking about are nerves. Nerves, if they are injured, can cause 5. _____ and pain. In the setting of prostate cancer, up to 60 percent of men after prostate cancer surgery may have 6. _____ incontinence and erectile 7. _____.

B. And we eventually discovered 8. _____ that were specifically labeling nerves. And when we made a 9. _____ of this, tagged with the 10. _____ and 11. _____ in the body of a mouse, their nerves literally glowed. You can see where they are.

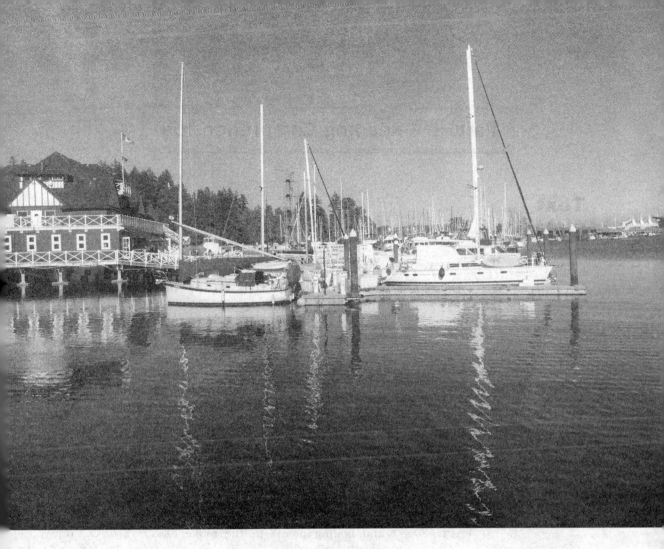

C. Basically, we've come up with a way to stain 12. _____ and color-code the
13. _____ field. This was a bit of a breakthrough. I think that it'll change the
way we do surgery. And we showed it to a lot of my colleagues. They said,
"Wow! I have patients who would benefit from this. I think that this will result in
my surgeries with a better 14. _____ and fewer 15. _____."

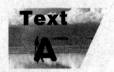

Diesel Oil Vapor Inhalation: Risk Factor for Heart Attack

Ahmadi M and Ahmadi R

Ⅰ. INTRODUCTION

GASOLINE is a liquid fuel intended for use in spark-ignition, internal combustion engines and the U. S. gasoline production in 2013 was the highest on record (API, 2013) and it is a blended product (i. e., mixture), which is not listed on the Toxic Substances Control Act (TSCA) Chemical Inventory. It is typically composed of hundreds of paraffinic, olefinic, naphthenic and aromatic hydrocarbons (generally referred to as PONA) refined from petroleum (crude oil) in the C4—C12 carbon-chain length range (API, 2008) and boiling points in the range of 30—220 ℃. In addition to the hydrocarbon base, gasoline also can contain a variety of blending components, such as oxygenates (e. g., alcohols, ethers). During gasoline manufacture, crude oil is fractionated, the fractions are chemically modified, and resulting refinery process "streams" are blended to meet specific physical and chemical property requirements (e. g., octane rating, sulfur limits, oxygen content, etc.). The 1990 amendments to the Clean Air Act (CAA) mandated the use of oxygenates in motor gasoline. In 1994, the U. S. Environmental Protection Agency (EPA) issued a final rule under the Act which added new health effects information and testing requirements to the Agency's existing registration requirements. As described in more detail in a companion paper (Henley et al. , 2014), requirements include inhalation exposures to evaporative emissions of the gasoline or additive in question. The health endpoints include assessments for standard subchronic toxicity, neurotoxicity, genotoxicity, immunotoxicity, developmental and reproductive toxicity, and chronic toxicity/

carcinogenicity. The results of chronic toxicity testing of gasoline and gasoline combined with MTBE have already been reported and reported elsewhere in this issue are the findings for genotoxicity, neurotoxicity, immunotoxicity, reproductive toxicity, and developmental toxicity testing in mice and rats. Key differences between whole gasoline and the vaporized gasoline are the significantly greater concentration of C4 and C5 constituents and depletion of C7—C12 aromatic constituents in the vapor condensate. The equilibrium vapor and vapor condensate are also less complex and have a lower average molecular weight and specific gravity. Human studies of both short- and long-term exposures to combustion emissions and ambient fine particulate air pollution have been associated with measures of genetic damage. Long-term epidemiologic studies have reported an increased risk of all causes of mortality, cardiopulmonary mortality, and lung cancer mortality associated with increasing exposures to air pollution. Adverse reproductive effects (e. g. ; risk for low birth weight) have also recently been reported in Eastern Europe and North America.

The contraction of invertebrate striated skeletal and cardiac muscle, is regulated by changes in the Ca^{2+} concentration inside the cell. These changes are sensed by the troponin (Tn) complex and transmitted to the other components of the contractile unit. The troponin complex is formed by three subunits, troponin C (TnC), troponin I (TnI), and troponin T (TnT). Tn C is an EF-hand protein that can bind four Ca^{2+} ions and is responsible for sensing the increase in calcium concentration. Two of its EF-hand sites, located in the C-domain, are high-affinity sites, capable of binding both Ca^{2+} and Mg^{2+}. These sites are occupied both during contraction and in the relaxed state. The other two EF-hand sites, located in the N-domain, are Ca^{2+}-specific and have lower affinity, being occupied when the intracellular Ca^{2+} levels rise during contraction, and empty in the relaxed state. This change in occupancy changes the interactions between TnC and TnI, and these conformational changes are transmitted to the rest of the thin filament, regulating muscle contraction. The only interaction between TnC and TnI is the structural interaction between the C-domain of TnC and the N-terminal region of TnI. When Ca^{2+} levels inside the cell rise, the N-domain of TnC interacts with the "switch" region of TnI (residues 116—131 in skeletal TnI), removing the interactions between TnI and actin and, consequently, the inhibition. The cardiac isoforms of TnC and TnI differ significantly from skeletal isoforms. In the cardiac isoform of TnC, Ca^{2+}-binding site I is naturally inactive and was found to undergo chemical exchange consistent with an equilibrium between "closed" and "open" forms.

II. MATERIAL AND METHODS

A. Animals

Adult Wistar rats weighting $200 \pm 30g$ were purchased and raised in our colony from an original stock of Pasteur institute (Tehran, Iran). The temperature was at 23 ± -2 ℃ and animals kept under a schedule of 12h light:12h darkness (light on at: 08: 00 a. m.) with free access to water and standard laboratory chow. This study was performed according to ethical guidelines relating to working with laboratory animals.

B. Protocol of Study

Male Wistar rats were randomly divided into control and groups exposed to diesel oil vapor for 1, 4 or 8h/day of 5 rats in each group. After 8 weeks, blood samples were obtained using cardiac puncture method. Following serum preparation, level of cardiac troponin was measured using immunoassay method.

C. Statistical Analysis

All values are presented as mean $\pm$ S. E. M. Statistical significance was evaluated by one-way analysis of variance (ANOVA) using SPSS 19. Differences with $P < 0.05$[①] were considered significant.

III. RESULTS

Table 1 and Figure 1 show the serum levels of Troponin C in male rats. The results indicated that serum level of cardiac troponin increased in rats exposed to diesel oil vapor for 4 and 8h/day compared to control rats ($P<0.001$ and $P<0.05$, respectively).

Group	Serum Troponin (ng/dl)	P
Control	1.92 ± 0.40	—
1h/day	2.06 ± 0.32	NS
4h/day	3.53 ± 0.18	<0.001
8h/day	3.00 ± 0.10	<0.05

TABLE 1

医学英语学术交流教程

Serum level of troponin C in control animals and rats exposed to diesel oil vapor for 1, 4 and 8 h/day. P values are versus control group. <u>NS indicates in significant difference</u> compared to control group.

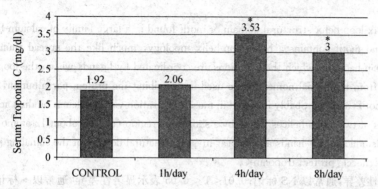

Fig. 1   Serum level of troponin C in control animals and rats exposed to diesel oil vapor for 1, 4 and 8h/day. * represents significant difference compared to control rats.

Ⅳ. DISCUSSION

Our study indicated that diesel oil vapor inhalation results in increased serum levels of troponin C.

Other studies have shown an association between air pollution and diseases. It has been suggested a possible association between chronic low level benzene exposure and increased risk of leukemia. It has also been shown that air pollution is associated with significant public health impacts, with cardiovascular disease being a prominent outcome. Studies also suggest that indoor air pollution from use of solid fuel is an important cause of acute coronary syndrome. However, some studies have shown that unleaded gasoline vapors did not produce evidence of developmental toxicity.

Ⅴ. CONCLUSION

Our findings show that exposure to diesel vapor for long period of time enhances serum cardiac troponin level which may indicate damage to heart.

ACKNOWLEDGMENT

This research has been done with the support of Islamic Azad University, Hamedan Branch, Hamedan, Iran. We appreciate all who helped us to exert the present study.

(1 107 words)

① The EF hand is a helix-loop-helix structural domain or motif found in a large family of calcium-binding proteins. The EF-hand motif contains a helix-loop-helix topology, much like the spread thumb and forefinger of the human hand, in which the Ca^{2+} ions are coordinated by ligands within the loop. The motif takes its name from traditional nomenclature used in describing the protein parvalbumin, which contains three such motifs and is probably involved in muscle relaxation via its calcium-binding activity. The EF-hand consists of two alpha helices linked by a short loop region (usually about 12 amino acids) that usually binds calciumions. EF-hands also appear in each structural domain of the signaling protein calmodulin and in the muscle protein troponin-C.

② P>0.05 表示无显著性差异,通常以 NS 标记;0.01<P<0.05 表示显著性差异,通常以 * 标记;P< 0.01 表示极显著性差异,通常以 * * 标记。

 Vocabulary

spark-ignition, internal combustion engines		火花点火式内燃机
Toxic Substance Control Act(TSCA)		［美］有毒物质管理法
paraffinic	[pærə'fɪnɪk]	adj. 石蜡族的
olefinic	[ɒlɪfɪ'nɪk]	adj. 烯烃的
naphthenic	[næf'θɪnɪk]	adj. 环烷烃的
aromatic	[ˌærə'mætɪk]	adj. 芳香烃的
hydrocarbons	[haɪdrə'kabənz]	n. ［化］碳氢化合物,烃
PONA	abbr. paraffin; olefin; naphthene; aromatic (test for petroleum octane rating 辛烷值) 链烷烃	
carbon chain length range		碳链长度范围
hydrocarbon base		烃类基质
oxygenate		v. 氧化
fractionate	['frækʃəneɪt]	v. (用分馏法等)分解
refinery process		精馏过程
mandate	['mændeɪt]	v. 授权;强制执行
evaporative emissions		蒸发性排放
in question		所说的,前述的,争议中的
carcinogenicity	[kɑsɪnəʊdʒə'nɪsəti]	n. 致癌力,致癌性
MTBE (methyl tert-butyl ether)		甲基叔丁基醚
depletion	[dɪ'pliʃən]	v. 消耗,用尽;耗减
ambient	['æmbɪənt]	adj. (产生轻松)氛围的;周围的,环境的
fine particulate air pollution		细颗粒物空气污染
mortality	[mɒr'tæləti]	n. 死亡数,死亡率;必死性,必死的命运

adverse	['ædvɜːs]	adj. 不利的；有害的；逆的；相反的
striated	['straɪeɪtɪd]	adj. 横纹的，有沟痕/线条的
Ca²⁺		n. 正2价的钙离子
cardiac troponin	['trɒpənɪn]	心肌肌钙蛋白
EF-hand		n. EF 手形结构（域）
intracellular	[ˌɪntrə'seljələ]	adj. [生]细胞内的
conformational change		构象改变
thin filament		细肌丝
residue	['rezɪdʊ]	n. 残余物，残渣，余渣
actin	['æktɪn]	n. 肌动蛋白
cardiac isoform		心肌亚型
chow		n. 食物
protocol	['prəʊtəkɒl]	n. 实验计划，医疗方案；协议，规程；草案；议定书
cardiac puncture method		心脏穿刺法
serum preparation		血清制备
immunoassay method		免疫法
mean ± S. E. M.		abbr. standard error of measurement 均数标准误
ANOVA		abbr. analysis of variance 方差/变量/离散分析
serum level		血清浓度水平
Ng/dl		abbr. microgram/deciliter 微克/分升
NS		nonsignificant difference compared to control group
benzene	['benziːn]	n. 苯
cardiovascular	[ˌkɑːdɪəʊ'væskjələ(r)]	adj. 心血管的

◆ Questions

1. Why is gasoline not listed on the Toxic Substances Control Act (TSCA) Chemical Inventory despite the fact that exposure to diesel vapor for a long period of time enhances serum cardiac troponin level which may indicate damage to heart?

2. What might be the reason why such oxygenates as alcohols and ethers are recommended and even forced to be added proportionally into gasoline?

3. What kind of ions' concentration is in charge of regulating the contraction of vertebrate striated skeletal and cardiac muscle at cellular level and what kind of protein can bind the ions?

4. What does mean ± S. E. M. indicate? If the difference probability value is 0.063,

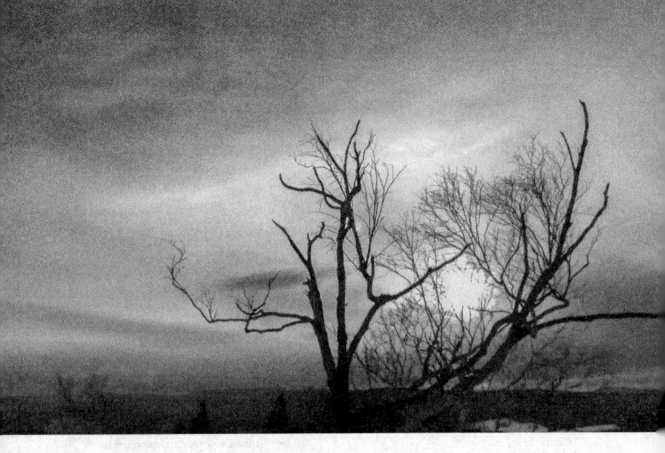

how should we treat the result of the study and what are the three typical symbols of the three common probabilities?

5. In the last paragraph of the passage, what do you think those significant public health impacts mean or include and what do they have in common medically?

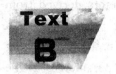

Heart Rate Variability Applied to Short-Term Cardiovascular Event Risk Assessment

Simao Paredes[1], Teresa Rocha[1], Paulo de Carvalho[2],
Jorge Henriques[2], Ramona Cabiddu[3], João Morais[4]

ABSTRACT

Cardiovascular disease (CVD) risk assessment is an important instrument to enhance the clinical decision in the daily practice as well as to improve the preventive health care promoting the transfer from the hospital to patient's home. Due to its importance, clinical guidelines recommend the use of risk scores to predict the risk of a cardiovascular disease event. Therefore, there are several well-known risk assessment tools, unfortunately they present some limitations. This work addresses this problem with two different methodologies: 1) combination of risk assessment tools based on fusion of Bayesian classifiers complemented with genetic algorithm optimization; 2) personalization of risk assessment through the creation of groups of patients that maximize the performance of each risk assessment tool. This last approach is implemented based on subtractive clustering applied to a reduced-dimension space. Both methodologies were developed to short-term CVD risk prediction for patients with Acute Coronary Syndromes without ST segment elevation (ACS-NSTEMI). Two different real patients' datasets were considered to validate the developed strategies: 1) San-ta Cruz Hospital, Portugal, N = 460 patients; 2) Leiria-Pombal Hospital Centre, Portugal, N = 99 patients. This work improved the performance in relation to current risk assessment tools reaching maximum values of sensitivity, specificity and geometric mean of, respectively, 80.0%, 82.9%, 81.5%. Besides this enhancement, the proposed methodologies allow the incorporation of new risk factors, deal with missing risk factors and avoid the selection of a single tool to be applied in the daily clinical practice. In spite of these achievements, the CVD risk assessment (patient stratification) should be improved. The incorporation of new risk factors recognized as clinically significant, namely parameters derived from heart rate variability (HRV), is introduced in this work. HRV is a strong and independent predictor of mortality in patients following acute myocardial infarction. The impact of HRV parameters in the characterization of coronary artery disease (CAD) patients will be conducted during hospitalization of these patients in the Leiria-Pombal Hospital Centre (LPHC).

Key words: CVD Risk Assessment; Knowledge Management; Management of Cardiovascular Diseases; Decision-Support Systems

1. Introduction

Coronary heart disease (CHD), approximately half of all cardiovascular disease (CVD) deaths, is the single most common cause of death in Europe.

European Heart Network supports that around 80% of CHD are preventable, which shows that the improvement of preventive health care can originate important benefits reducing the incidence of cardiovascular diseases.

Therefore, preventive health care assumes a critical importance in the present health care context. It is the key aspect in reducing the social and economic costs directly originated by cardiovascular diseases. In fact, it is commonly accepted that current health care paradigm has to move from reactive care towards preventive care, reducing the amount of in hospital care. Health telemonitoring systems are essential to achieve this target, as they allow the remote monitoring of patients who are in different locations away from the health care provider. This remote monitoring is more challenging to the care provider, as the reliability/quality of the clinical decision must be guaranteed in order to optimize therapy.

The CVD risk assessment, i. e., the evaluation of the probability of occurrence of an event (death, myocardial infarction, hospitalization, disease development, etc.) gives the patient's past and current exposure to risk factors, assuming great importance in this remote health monitoring. It contributes in providing the patient's health development as well as generating alarms. In this way, a correct CVD risk assessment helps clinical professionals to identify the best treatment to each patient as well as to motivate the patient increasing the treatment compliance with the corresponding health benefits (patient seen as a co-producer of health).

Additionally, clinical guidelines recommend the use of risk scores in the daily clinical practice to predict the risk of a cardiovascular disease event. This assessment contributes in helping medical professionals in managing the patient population. Actually, physicians gather more information to identify the patients that need urgent hospitalization, those that need urgent review of respective care plans (lack of treatment, over treatment situations ...) and those that correspond with the expected condition.

As a result, it is clinically recognized that the research and development of practical and accurate CV risk assessment tools are of vital importance. In this context, several risk assessment tools were developed to assess the probability of occurrence of a CVD event within a certain period of time. Two types of risk may be calculated: absolute risk, i. e., probability of developing a CVD event over a given period of time (e. g. 10 years), and a relative risk, i. e., risk of someone developing a CVD event that has risk factors compared to an individual of the same age and sex who does not. Moreover, available risk assessment tools differ on the assessed period of time (short-term [months]/long-term[years]), predicted events (death/ non-fatal), disease (coronary artery disease, heart failure, etc.), risk factors, patient condition (ambulatory patients, hospitalized patients, cardiac transplant candidates, etc.).

In spite of their relevance, these risk assessment tools exhibit important drawbacks: 1) may present some lack of performance; 2) ignore the information provided by other risk assessment tools that were previously developed; 3) consider (each individual tool) a limited number of risk factors; 4) have difficulty in coping with missing risk factors; 5) do not allow the incorporation of additional clinical knowledge; 6) do not assure the clinical interpretability of the respective parameters; 7) impose a selection of a standard tool to be applied in the clinical practice.

This work addresses the identified weaknesses with two different methodologies: 1) combination of risk assessment tools (fusion of naïve Bayes classifiers complemented with genetic algorithm optimization); 2) personalization of risk assessment (creation of groups of patients based on subtractive clustering applied to a reduced-dimension space).

Two main hypotheses support the first approach: 1) it is possible to create a common representation of individual risk assessment tools; and 2) it is possible to combine individual models. The main goal is to integrate several sources of information (risk assessment tools) to defeat the identified limitations. Though, current risk assessment tools are diversely represented [8—10], which does not facilitate their integration/combination. Therefore, a common representation must be created verifying some requirements: 1) simplicity; 2) ability to incorporate new risk factors (empirical clinical knowledge); 3) clinical interpretability; and 4) ability to deal with missing risk factors. The creation of a flexible framework based on the combination of available knowledge, is the basis of the second hypothesis. According to various authors an ensemble of classifiers is often more accurate than any of the respective single classifiers. Thus, there are several methods to implement model's combination which can be organized in two main categories: 1) model output combination; and 2) model parameter/ data fusion. The former includes the voting (e. g. , voting, weighted voting, dynamic voting, bagging algorithms, boosting algorithms, etc.) and selection methods (e. g. , information criteria, cross-validation variants, dynamic selection, etc.) [11, 12]. Model parameter/data fusion implements a direct combination of the parameters of individual models [13,14]. The approach proposed in this work is included in this last category and explores the particular features of Bayesian inference mechanism. This framework also permits the implementation of optimization methodologies to increase the CVD risk prediction performance.

The second methodology, personalization of risk assessment, addresses the problem of the low performance exhibited by the current risk assessment tools when applied to the general population. The methodology is based on the evidence that risk assessment tools perform differently among different populations. Thus, the main hypothesis that supports this methodology can be stated as: if the patients are properly grouped (clustered) it would be possible to find the best classifier for each group.

The two methodologies were applied to three (GRACE, TIMI, PURSUIT) well-accepted risk assessment tools. The validation phase was supported by two real ACS-NSTEMI patient testing datasets: i) Santa Cruz Hospital, Lisbon/Portugal, N = 460 patients; ii) LeiriaPombal Hospital Centre, Portugal, N = 99.

In spite of these achievements, the CVD risk assessment

(patient stratification) should be improved. The possible incorporation of new risk factors recognized as clinically significant, namely parameters derived from heart rate variability (HRV), is introduced in this work. In fact, HRV is a strong and independent predictor of mortality in patients following acute myocardial infarction.

The paper is organized as follows: Section II presents the developed methodologies. In Section III some results of the validation procedure are discussed. Section IV depicts the incorporation of the heart rate variability parameters in the CVD risk assessment. The main conclusions are derived.

2. Methodology

Figure 1 presents the developed strategies. These methodologies were further detailed in previous publications of this research team [16,17].

2.1 Combination of Individual Tools

The implementation of this approach is composed of two main phases: 1) common representation of individual risk assessment tools based on naïve Bayes classifier; 2) a combination scheme that exploits the probabilistic nature of naïve-Bayes inference mechanism complemented with an optimization based on genetic algorithms (GA).

2.1.1 Common Representation of Individual Tools

Current individual risk scores (risk assessment tools) are diversely represented (equations/scores/charts) which hinder their combination. To allow the fusion (combination) of these risk scores a common representation is created. The classifier selected to implement this common representation is the naïve Bayes classifier as it presents some important features: 1) simplicity; 2) ability to deal with missing risk factors; and 3) interpretability. Its inference mechanism assumes that observations (attributes) are conditionally independent, given the value of hypothesis C:

$$P(C \mid x) = P(C \mid X_1, \dots, X_p) = \alpha P(C) \prod_{i=1}^{P} P(X_i \mid C) \qquad (1)$$

The term $P(C \mid x)$ is the probability that the hypothesis is correct (e. g. , the risk is high) given a set of attributes $x = [X_1, \dots, X_p]$ (e. g. , demographic data, clinical examination, laboratory measurements, etc.). $P(C)$ gives the prevalence of each risk level（a priori probability）and $P(X \mid C)$ expresses the probability of the observation X given the value of class of risk C (likelihood)，α is a normalization constant.

The process of representing a specific individual risk assessment tool as a naïve Bayes classifier can be systematized as follows: 1) a training dataset is generated，N instances $\mathbf{x} = [X_1, \ldots, X_p]$ composed of p attributes; 2) each instance is applied to the risk assessment tool in order to obtain a complete labeled dataset $J = \{(\mathbf{x}_1, c_1), \ldots, (\mathbf{x}_N, c_N)\}$; and 3) based on J and through the maximum likelihood estimation method，the naïve Bayes classifier that resembles the behavior of that specific risk assessment tool is derived. The probability $P(C)$ results directly from distribution of the class values (low risk/high risk patients).

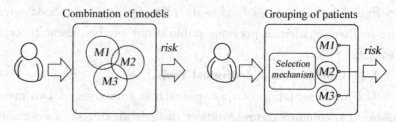

Figure 1   Proposed methodologies

2.1.2 Individual Models Parameters' Weighted Average

The Equation（2）implements the proposed combination scheme，where it is possible to assign different weights for the individual Bayesian models.

$$P(C) = \sum_{j=1}^{l} P(C_j) \times \frac{w_j}{\Gamma} \quad whee \ \Gamma = \sum_{j=1}^{l} w_j$$

$$P(X_i \mid C) = \sum_{j=1}^{b} P(X_i^j \mid C_j) \times \frac{w_j}{\theta} \ whee \ \theta = \sum_{j=1}^{b} w_j \quad (2)$$

Value l is the number of individual models，b is the number of individual models that contain the attribute X_i，C_j denotes each individual model，w_j is the weight of model j.

An optimization based on GA can be performed. The GA focuses on the $P(X_i \mid C)$，$P(C)$ that are the parameters of the global model originated through the combination method. The optimization is performed in the neighbourhood of the initial values and through a multi-objective approach where sensitivity and specificity should be maximized. A detailed approach to this optimization procedure can be found on.

医学英语学术交流教程

2.2　Personalization Based on Grouping of Patients

This second methodology was developed to enhance the performance of the risk prediction when compared to the one obtained with current risk assessment tools. It is based on the hypothesis that it is possible to select the most appropriate current risk assessment tool for a specific group of patients.

This methodology is composed of two main phases: 1) grouping of patients; and 2) identification of risk tools. Grouping of patients is supported on a dimension reduction step as it facilitates clustering; it avoids the heterogeneity (continuous, Boolean, etc.) of risk factors and it assures the uniformization of each patient's data (same scale). A non-linear mapping is implemented directly supported on the outputs of the selected set of risk assessment tools. Thus, all instances $\mathbf{x}_i = [x_1^i \dots x_P^i]^T \in \mathbf{X}_{P \cdot N}$, that correspond to the N patients are mapped into $y_i \in \mathbf{Y}_{Q \cdot N}$, $i = 1, \dots, N$ where $y_q i$ denotes the output of tool q to classify the patient i. Then, clustering is applied through subtractive clustering. Patients are grouped, based on the outputs of the risk tools $\mathbf{Y}_{Q \cdot N}$, in order to create K disjoint groups (clusters) of patients with similar characteristics.

The second phase is the identification of risk assessment tools, where the performance of the several individual tools is assessed within each cluster. This allows that each cluster be assigned to the tool that presents the best performance. The final classification of a particular patient that belongs to a given cluster corresponds to the classification obtained with the individual tool that has the best performance with patients from that cluster.

3.　Results

The two developed methodologies were applied to coronary artery disease patients (secondary prevention/short term) (Table 1).

The three risk assessment tools (TIMI, PURSUIT, GRACE) were selected as they are the most well accepted/known CVD risk assessment tools specific for CAD patients.

Two testing ACS-NSTEMI real patient datasets were applied in the validation procedure: 1) Santa Cruz hospital with N = 460 patients. The event rate of combined end-point (death/myocardial infarction) is 7.2%. 2) Leiria-Pombal Hospital Centre with N = 99 patients with an endpoint rate of 5.1%.

The training dataset was created $\mathbf{x}^i = [x_1^i \dots x^i p]$ for all i; $1 \leqslant$

$i \leqslant N$, with $N=1000$, based on the approach proposed in.

Table 1   Short-term risk assessment models

Model	Event	Time	Prev.	Risk Factors
GRACE[10]	D MI	6 m	Sec.	Age, SBP, CAAHR, Cr, STD, ECM, CHF
PURSUIT[9]	D MI	30 d	Sec.	Age, Sex, SBP, CCS, HR, STD, ERL, HF
TIMI[8]	MI UR	14d	Sec.	Age, STD, ECM, KCAD, AS, AG, RF

D: Death; **MI**: Myocardial Infarction; **UR**: Urgent revasc. ; **m**: months; **d**: days; **S**: Secondary Prevention; **Cr**—Creatinine, **HR**—Heart Rate, **CAA**—Cardiac Arrest at Admission, **CHF**—Congestive Heart Failure, **STD**—ST Segment Depression, **ECE**—Elevated Cardiac Markers/Enzymes, **KCAD**—Known CAD, **ERL**—Enrolment (MI/UA), **HF**—Heart Failure, **CCS**—Angina classification, **AS**—Use of aspirin in the previous 7 days, **AG**—2 or more angina events in past 24 hrs, **RF**—3 or more cardiac risk factors.

3.1   Combination of Individual Tools

Table 2 contains the comparison of the Bayesian global model with the individual risk assessment tools as well as with the voting model (based on the outputs of the three individual risk assessment tools).

Table 3 presents the results obtained after the optimization procedure based on GA operation.

Considering the obtained results in table, the optimization improved the capability of the global model to predict the risk. However, there were some test cases where the combination methodology did not achieve an improvement of the performance, namely of the specificity value.

3.2   Personalization Based on Grouping of Patients

This methodology was applied to the Santa Cruz hospital dataset (combined endpoint, D/MI), based on the same risk tools (TIMI, PURSUIT, GRACE). The first step was the dimensionality reduction from the original $P = 16$ risk factors to $Q = 3$ outputs of the risk tools. The clusters were created and the performance of each tool in each cluster was assessed.

This strategy achieved a higher sensitivity than all the individual tools (the best individual sensitivity is 60.8% while the sensitivity for the proposed strategy is 72.9%) (Table 4). It did not reduce the specificity, which shows the potential of this approach to improve the risk prediction.

More detailed results obtained with the validation of these two methodologies, can be found on [16,17].

4. Final Considerations

4.1 Ongoing Research

In spite of the performance enhancements, there are some research directions that must be pursued to improve the CVD risk assessment. The fusion of the two developed methodologies must be further explored (personalization). Furthermore, the flexibility of the combination methodology (Bayesian global model) allows the incorporation of parameters recognized as clinically significant to improve risk assessment, namely the heart rate variability (HRV).

Heart Rate Variability

Heart rate variability is an ECG derived signal consisting in the oscillation in the interval between consecutive heart beats.

Table 2　Performances comparison—Santa cruz, (D/MI)

	%	GRACE	PURSUIT	TIMI	ByG	Vot
Orig.	SE	60.6	42.4	33.3	60.6	48.5
	SP	74.9	74.2	73.5	67.0	75.6
	Gmean	67.3	56.0	49.4	63.4	60.6
Boot samples $n = 1000$	SE	60.8 (60.2; 61.3)	42.4 (41.9; 43.1)	33.5 (33.0; 34.0)	60.6 (60.1; 61.3)	48.6 (48.0; 49.2)
	SP	74.9 (74.8; 75.1)	74.2 (74.1; 74.3)	73.6 (73.5; 73.7)	67.0 (66.9; 67.2)	75.6 (75.5; 75.8)
	Gmean	67.3 (67.0; 67.6)	55.8 (55.5; 56.2)	49.3 (48.9; 49.7)	63.6 (63.3; 63.9)	60.3 (60.0; 60.7)

SE: Sensitivity; SP: Specificity; D: Death; MI: Myocardial Infarction; (—; —) = 95% CI; ByG—Bayesian Global Model, Vot—Voting

Table 3　Performances comparison

		Santa Cruz 30 days/D/MI		Santa Cruz 30 days/D		Santo André 30 days/D	
		ByG	ByGAO	ByG	ByGAO	ByG	ByGAO
Orig.	SE	60. 6	72. 7	61. 5	76. 9	80. 0	80. 0
	SP	67. 0	69. 1	65. 7	70. 7	67. 0	82. 9
	Gmean	63. 4	70. 9	63. 5	73. 7	73. 2	81. 5
Boot Samples $n = 1000$	SE	60. 6 (60. 1; 61. 3)	72. 9 (72. 4; 73. 4)	61. 6 (60. 7; 62. 5)	77. 3 (76. 5; 78. 0)	80. 3 (78. 9; 81. 5)	79. 8 (78. 6; 81. 0)
	SP	67. 0 (66. 9; 67. 2)	69. 1 (69. 0; 69. 2)	65. 8 (65. 6; 65. 9)	70. 6 (70. 5, 70. 8)	66. 8 (66. 4; 67. 2)	83. 8 (83. 3; 84. 2)
	Gmean	63. 6 (63. 3; 63. 9)	70. 9 (70. 6; 71. 1)	63. 1 (62. 7; 63. 6)	73. 6 (73. 3; 74. 0)	72. 3 (71. 5; 73. 1)	80. 9 (80. 0; 81. 6)

ByG—Bayesian Global Model; **ByG AO**—Bayesian Global Model after Optimization

Table 4　Performances comparison—Santa cruz（Death/MI）

	%	GRACE	PURSUIT	TIMI	Groups
Boot. samples $n = 1000$	SE	60. 8 (60. 2; 61. 3)	42. 4 (41. 9;43. 1)	33. 5 (33. 0; 34. 0)	72. 9 (72. 6; 73. 5)
	SP	74. 9 (74. 8; 75. 1)	74. 2 (74. 1;74. 3)	73. 6 (73. 5; 73. 7)	74. 9 (74. 8; 75. 1)

Cardiac rhythmical activity is controlled by the auto-nomic nervous system（ANS）where the sympathetic system（arousal/activation）and parasympathetic system（inhibition）are the key elements. A significant correlation between autonomic functionality and CV mortality is documented. Increased HRV reflects a healthy ANS that is able to respond to changes in the environmental circumstances. By contrast, decreased HRV is a marker of ANS inflexibility, which may precede more systemic problems.

Depressed HRV has been reported in several CVD, including coronary artery disease（CAD）and heart failure. Actually, HRV is a strong and independent predictor of mortality in CAD patients（after MI）. HRV is depressed in these patients, with a reduction in the total power of the signal, presenting some parameters that indicate a prevalence of sympathetic activation, which may lead to cardiac electrical instability. Thus, HRV parameters (time domain, frequency domain) should be explored as quantitative markers of ANS activity, as they are significantly correlated with all-cause mortality, cardiac death, and arrhythmic death [20,22].

HRV is usually assessed with two types of recordings: 1) short-term (e. g. , 5 minutes); 2) long-term (~24 hours). Although the latter is a stronger risk predictor, HRV assessed from short recordings also provides useful prognostic information. Ideally, HRV parameters should be assessed within one week after MI. However, these parameters are significant mortality predictors even when measured after that period.

Current risk assessment tools do not include HRV parameters. However, there are several HRV derived parameters that can potentially be applied to improve the CVD risk assessment. The flexibility of the developed Bayesian global model solves this problem, as it allows a straightforward integration of additional knowledge/new risk factors.

This is the main focus of the ongoing research: the selection and incorporation of HRV parameters in order to improve risk assessment and consequently the patients' stratification. The incorporation mechanism is assured by the developed combination methodology however the selection of the specific HRV parameters must be care-fully considered.

Time domain parameters may include: 1) *HRV mean*, the average value of RR interbeat intervals; 2) *HRV SDNN* the normal-to-normal (NN) intervals standard deviation; 3) *HRV RMSSD* the square root of the mean squared differences of successive NN intervals; 4) *HRV NN* 50 the number of interval differences of successive NN intervals greater than 50 ms; and 5) *HRV pNN* 50 the proportion of NN50 considering the total of NN intervals.

In the frequency domain, three main spectral components can be identified: the very low frequency (VLF: 0.01—0.04 Hz), the low frequency (LF: 0.04—0.15 Hz) and the high frequency components (HF: 0.15—0.4 Hz). Changes in the LF and the HF components reflect sympathetic and parasympathetic activities, and their ratio (LF/HF) is considered as a marker of the sympathovagal balance controlling the heart rate. A different energy distribution was observed in MI patients, VLF components are responsible for the main amount while a minor part is assigned to HF components. The correlation between these components and specific conditions must be further investigated to obtain the required data to perform the incorporation in the global framework. Spectral analysis must be conducted on the HRV signals obtained from the ECG recordings performed on CAD patients.

Non-linear phenomena are also involved in HRV as cardiac activity is also regulated by intrinsically non-linear mechanisms. Some non-linear parameters can be identified such as 1/f slope of Fourier spectra, Sample Entropy, Lempel-Ziv Complexity.

The impact of HRV parameters in the characterization of CAD patients will be conducted during hospitalization of these patients in LPHC. An integrated clinical platform, integrating the developed algorithms, will be implemented. In addition to the information obtained from the hospital information system, ECG (Holter) signals will be collected to derive the HRV parameters.

5. Conclusion

The two developed methodologies improved the performance of risk assessment when compared to the one achieved by the current risk assessment tools. Moreover, the combination methodology allows important features such as the ability to deal with missing risk factors as well as the incorporation of new risk factors. However, we believe that the incorporation of the Heart Rate Variability parameters can significantly improve the risk assessment/patient stratification.

6. Acknowledgement

This work was partially financed by iCIS (CENTRO-07-ST24-FEDER-002003) and by Cardiorisk (PTDC/EEI-SII/2002/2012).

(3780 words)

※ The text is extracted from *Engineering*, 2013, 5, 237—243, published online October 2013. (http://www.scirp.org/journal/eng)

Practice 1

Clinical Inquiry—Operating Room

Vocabulary

anaesthesia	[ˌænəsˈθiːzɪə]	*n.* 麻醉 loss of sensitivity to pain in all or a part of the body for medical reasons.
consent	[kənˈsent]	*n.* /*v.* 同意，允许 agreement on an opinion or course of action
(the)undersigned	[ˌʌndəˈsaɪnd]	*n.* 签名人，署名人 somebody whose signature appears on the document being read
immediate family		直系亲属 nearest in time, space, or relationship
enema	[ˈenəmə]	*n.* 灌肠 a medical treatment in which liquid is forced into a person's intestines through their anus
anus	[ˈeɪnəs]	*n.* 肛门 the opening at the lower end of the alimentary canal through which feces are released
soapsuds solution	[ˈsəʊpˌsʌdz səˈluːʃ(ə)n]	*n.* 肥皂溶液 the white bubbles that are formed when you mix soap with water
distension	[dɪˈstenʃ(ə)n]	*n.* 扩张，膨胀 being distended, expanding because of pressure from inside
expel	[ɪkˈspel]	*v.* 排出，排放 to push or drive something out with force

Using Lay Terms in Explanations

Explanations should be given in words the patients can understand, avoiding medical terms. Using lay terms—words familiar to people without medical knowledge—can help patients understand explanations. e. g. :

Medical Terms	Lay Terms
1. anaesthesia	state of being unable to feel
2. enema	injection of liquid into the rectum
3. distension	swelling
4. expel	let go

Sample Dialogue

Nurse (N): We are going to do the operation on you tomorrow. I hope you won't worry.

Patient (P): I will try not to, but will it hurt?

N: We'll give you an aesthesia. If you feel any pain during the operation, just let me know. Have you hand in your consent yet?

P: How should I write it?

N: "I (name) the undersigned have requested and consented to a certain operation. " That's all. We need the seal of your embassy and the signature of your immediate family on the consent form. OK, now, I'd like to shave off the hair around the operation.

P: I have never been in a hospital before. I'm so scared.

N: There is nothing to worry about. The doctor who will operate on you is very experienced and considerate. If you have any discomfort during the operation, please don't hesitate to tell him. I'll give you an enema tonight. After that please don't take any food or water before the operation.

P: How do you do it? Does it hurt?

N: I'll insert a rubber tube into your anus and let the soapsuds solution flow into your rectum. Please let me know if you feel distension. I'll stop the flowing. Hold it for several minutes before you expel it. That may produce a better result.

...

N: The operation went very well. Please turn from side to side every two or three hours.

P: I only feel mild pain. I don't think a pain-killer is necessary. /The pain is very severe. I can't stand it. Please give me a pain-killer at once.

N: I'll help you get up. You can try walking around the room or corridor.

P: I think I'm quite all right now.

Practice 2 ▮▮▮

International Conference
—Acceptant Speech and Congratulations

 Useful Expressions for Acceptant Speech

1. I dedicate this award to all the people who have devoted their life to diabetic research and millions of people who still suffer diabetes today.

2. Ladies and gentlemen, all my colleagues and friends: I'm so surprised. I can hardly believe it.

3. I don't know what to say. My dream came true.

4. My prayers have been answered. I thank God for my very good luck.

5. First, thank you all, I appreciate this so much.

6. I will treasure this moment for a long time. It feels just great, and it's like I'm floating on air.

7. It means a lot to me. However, we all did our best, and we tried as hard as we could. We are all winners.

8. I've learned two valuable lessons from this award: "Believe in your potential. " and "Hard work really does pay off!" This is my advice to everybody. If I can win this, anyone can do it!

9. This award strengthens my resolve. Finally, prizes are material, and awards come and go, but this memory will last forever.

10. A final thanks to the judges. I'm flattered to be selected.

11. Hi, everyone! It is a great honor for access to this award for medical research. I am very touched.

12. I'm stuck for words at this moment. I have treasured the opportunity and thoroughly enjoyed my time with all of you, both my friends and fellow colleagues. Without you, I wouldn't have achieved this much. And I am confident that your support will add greatly to my career future. Thank you.

 Useful Expressions for Congratulations

1. Congratulations! Your honor brings to all of us.

2. Congratulations on your success!

3. Congratulations! Earning the award is an achievement of note, and I hope you are

feeling proud and happy, as you deserve.

4. Congratulations on all that you've accomplished. Good luck in all that you'll achieve.

5. Congratulations on your achievements in cancer research! It must be a wonderful feeling to have reached this milestone, and I envy you the opportunities that lie ahead.

6. I wish you every success in the future. You are worthy of success.

7. You have now satisfied a lifelong ambition! My heartiest congratulations and best wishes for every future success.

Activities and Role-play (inviting students to improvise and act it out)

Practice 3 ‖‖‖‖
Oral English for Culture and on Social Occasions—Buddhism

Buddhism in China

Buddhism is practiced in many countries and cultures throughout the world. Mahayana Buddhism has played a significant role in China and it has a long and rich history.

As Buddhism grew in the country, it adapted to and influenced the Chinese culture and a number of schools were developed. And yet, it wasn't always good to be a Buddhist in China as some found out under the persecution of various rulers.

Introduction of Buddhism

The coming of Buddhism to China from India was a great event in the development of Chinese culture and of Buddhism itself. After a long period of assimilation, it established itself as a major system of thought as well as a religious practice, contributing greatly to the enrichment of Chinese philosophy and exercising and enduring influence on the Chinese popular religion and on the mind and character of the Chinese people. Indeed, it becomes one of the Three Pillars of the traditional culture of China.

Buddhism was firstly introduced into the region inhabited by the Han people around the 1st century. It is said that in the year 2 BC, Yi Cun, an emissary of Dayuezhi Kingdom (an ancient mid-Asian country established by a strong Chinese minority originally living in northern China and later moved to the west), went to Chang'an (today's Xi'an City) to impact Buddhist sutras to a Chinese doctor Jing Lu. And this is the first record about the introduction of Buddhism into China.

There is another saying that during the reign of the Indian King Asoka (272—226 BC), 18 Indians visited China's Xianyang City during the reign of Emperor Qin Shihuang. In the year 250 BC, King Asoka convoked the third conference and after the conference, Dade was sent to spread Buddhism to other countries, including China.

Status of Chinese Buddhism

The feature of Chinese Buddhism lies in the coexistence of Mahayana Buddhism and Hinayana Buddhism as well as the concomitance of Exoteric and Esoteric Buddhism. Buddhism was initiated in India, developed in China and further expanded to Japan and Korea. However, Buddhist doctrinal classification itself never played any crucial role in Indian Buddhism as it did in China. Indian Buddhists were threatened by the values and socio-political structures of the Indian society dominated by Hinduism and Islam and vanished between 9th century and 10th century in India while Buddhism was developed rapidly in China so that China became the true homeland of Buddhism all over the world. Particularly worth mentioning is that Buddhism integrated Chinese culture and developed some branches with Chinese characteristics, like Tibetan Buddhism, Theravada Buddhism.

During the Wei and Jin Dynasties (220—420) the influence of Buddhism spread widely. During the Southern and Northern Dynasties(420—589) the ruling classes further helped the spread of Buddhism by building temples and monasteries, translating Buddhist sutras and constructing grottoes, and many famous monks, scholars and teachers emerged. By the Sui and Tang Dynasties (581—907), Buddhism reached its apex of popularity and splendors, and different sects of Buddhism had been formed in China. Over a long period, Buddhism gradually took root in the feudal society of China, intermingling with Confucian and Taoist thoughts. It had a strong popular appeal and its ideas made a notable impact on Chinese philosophy, literature and art.

The Influence to China

Since introduced to China, Buddhism has influenced to Chinese culture and Chinese people's life. Many frescoes, sculptures, grottoes, philosophy, literature greatly relate to Buddhism culture. To some extent, Buddhism makes a great contribution to Chinese culture.

Top Buddhist Destinations in China
Shanxi Province

It is where the sacred Mount Wutai located. At an altitude of around 3000 m, Mount Wutai is known as the residence of the Bodhisattva Manjusri, and the number one holy place of Buddhism in China. There were 300 temples in its heyday, but only 47 of them are left today, with a wealth of collections of Buddhist art works, classics, Buddhist sculptures and other heritages. Other famous Buddhist shrines in Shanxi include Yungang Grottoes in Datong, the Hanging Monastery, and Yingxian Wooden Pagoda.

Tibet

As one of the best-known Buddhist sanctuaries in the world, Tibet boasts many holy temples, mountains, caves and lakes. Lasa is the holy city of Tibetan Buddhism, while Potala Palace is the Tibetan Buddhist center. Built in the Tang Dynasty, Potala Palace is a treasure house of Tibetan Buddhist culture and art, and Tibetan architectural complex. Other famous Buddhist temples in Lasa include Jokhang Temple, Sera Monastery, Drepung Monastery, Gandan Monastery.

Mount Emei

The residence of Samantabhadra Bodhisattva, Mount Emei is one of the four holy Buddhist mountains in China. 30 of the over 100 temples are left and well preserved today, including the famous Wannian Temple, Baoguo Temple and Qingyin Pavilion. The beautiful scenery, splendid Buddhist culture, magnificent Buddha statues and century-old architectures make Mount Emei a UNESCO World Natural and Cultural Heritage site, together with the Leshan Giant Buddha (50 km away from Mt. Emei).

Mount Putuo

100 sea miles east of Jiaodong Bay, Hangzhou, holy Putuo Mountain (where Arya Avalokiteshvara practiced Buddhism) is hidden on the Zhoushan Islands, and surrounded by the sea. Every year numerous Buddhists and believers make a pilgrimage to Mount Putuo to study Buddhism, burn incense and pray.

Mount Jiuhua

Legend has that Ksitigarbha Bodhisattva used to practice Buddhism on Mount Jiuhua. 20 km southwest of Qingyang Town, Anhui Province, it is a branch range of Yellow Mountain, with 99 towering peaks. Mount Jiuhua is not only famous for its profound Buddhist culture, but also the breathtaking mountain views.

White Horse Temple in Luoyang, Henan Province

The first Buddhist temple in China, it was built in the year of 68 during the East Han Dynasty, when Buddhism began to be introduced to China. The original architecture was magnificent, but partly destroyed in history.

Famen Temple in Xi'an

Famen Temple was the royal temple in the Tang Dynasty and has been a Buddhist holy land by keeping the finger bones of Sakyamuni.